SOUVENIRS OF SUFFERING

SOUVENIRS OF SUFFERING

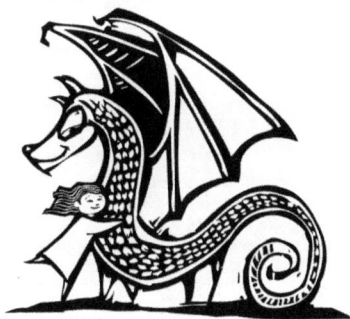

DAZHONI GREEN

Prairie Stone Press, Minneapolis, MN
Copyright © 2019 Dazhoni Green
Cover art and illustrations by Tim Green
All rights reserved.

ISBN: 978-1-7332930-0-6

In loving memory of Uncle Lonnie and
Uncle Bruce.

Dedicated to the children
I met along the way who were later
given their angel wings.

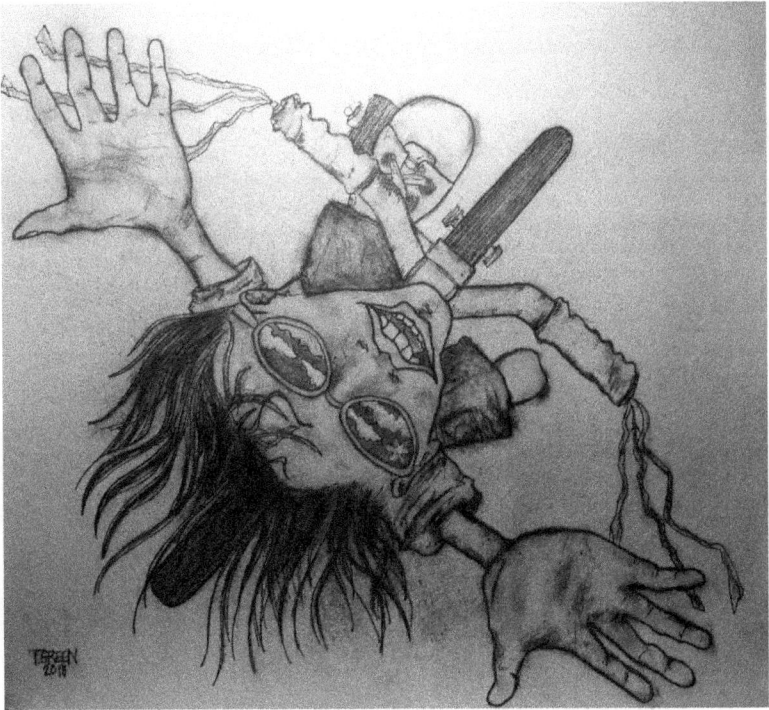

Foreword

This book chronicles the suffering, uncertainty and ultimate triumph of a child overcoming brain cancer. Facing unrelenting illness, before and after surgery, Dazhoni endures each step of her journey through the support of family members, friends, and countless others who held out loving hands. This is the story of crossing the threshold from childhood to the broader world of faith, gratitude and empathy.

Contents

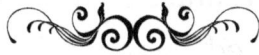

Something Good

"ARGH!"

In the blink of an eye, I was looking at the plastic container of potato salad that was now a gooey mess all over the counter, the floor, and my fist. My mom and sister were staring at me open mouthed from the dining room table.

I took off in the direction of my room, stubbing my toe on a chair leg, the shooting pain making me even more upset. I yelled again as I tore through our living room and down the hallway.

"When will you learn to control your temper?" I heard Mom say before I slammed my bedroom door shut. I knew she was about to scold me; she had just told me to let her try to open the container when I had begun to get frustrated.

My temper. It was my fatal flaw. I hadn't been angry like this my whole life; it happened after my parents' divorce about a year and a half ago. I missed Dad and how our lives used to be. Feeling sorry for myself, I sank down with my back against the door and kicked aside my Pokémon cards that were scattered across the carpet. This was how I sat when I didn't want my mom or bratty sister barging in.

We had just moved to this little townhouse in Hawley, Minnesota, a few months ago. We used to live in an even smaller town about a forty-minute drive away. Mom was having a hard time finding work, and the big old house in Rothsay was too cold and too hard to manage without Dad around to keep things working.

There was another reason why we had moved. Me. I had gotten into trouble at school, fighting with kids during recess. And there were also the days I would kick and scream, refusing to go to school at all. Mom hoped that I just needed a fresh start at a new school, a new town, and new kids.

I was doing okay, so far. No more fighting. But I didn't have anyone to talk to during lunchtime, or anyone to play with during recess. Ever since my parents separated, it's been hard to make friends.

Suddenly I remembered! Something good. I reached over and grabbed a shoulder strap on my backpack and pulled it towards me. Unzipping the largest pocket, I dug my hand in. Got it! Pulling out a folded piece of paper, I jumped to my feet.

No longer angry, I skipped out the door and through the hallway. "Hey, Mom! Guess what! I'm invited to a birthday party!" I couldn't wait to tell her about the new friend I had made at school. She was in a different fifth grade class than me, but I often ran into her in the hallway.

"Look!" I unfolded the invitation as I made it to the kitchen. Maybe this was the start for me getting my life back to normal, the way it was before the divorce.

"For Ariel's birthday next Saturday, we'll all be going out to eat and then shopping at Claire's and the mall! Ariel said her mom would pick me up and then drop me off home."

I felt like jumping up and down when I noticed Mom holding a rag and looking up at me. She had just finished cleaning up the mess I had made and I felt bad.

"Is there a number I can call?" she finally said.

"Yeah." I pointed to the bottom of the paper. Although she was probably still upset with me, she smiled. I knew she was happy for me. I had finally made a friend, and I finally had something to look forward to.

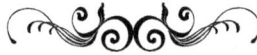

A Birthday Party

How can this be happening to me?

I tried denying it until I couldn't any longer. It was going to happen. And of all the kids in the world who weren't afraid of throwing up, it had to be happening to me. I ignored the headache at the restaurant and then the burps when I piled back into the van, but I couldn't ignore the sick feeling in the pit of my stomach. It climbed up my throat as I followed the group of girls through the sliding doors at the mall. I was going to throw up!

My brain went into panic mode. *Should I tell Ariel's mom? Will this ruin Ariel's birthday? Will I make it to the toilet?* This was a nightmare!

Burp. All the spit in my mouth was gone.

The moment I spotted a restroom off to my right, I broke away from the birthday girl and the rest of the group.

Ariel's mom turned and looked at me. "Are you all right, hon?"

I wasn't going to ruin the afternoon for everyone else. "I'll catch up with you guys," I choked, giving her a thumbs up. I pushed the heavy door open, disappearing inside.

Burp. That one reached my mouth.

I ran into the only open stall. Telling myself not to cry, I knelt down by the toilet.

How did this happen? Was it the burger I had just eaten? How did I get so sick so fast?

When I lifted the seat, I saw yellow stains on the rim. I closed my eyes and plugged my ears. No way was I going to watch this. All I could hear were my thoughts and my beating heart.

Throwing up was my biggest, most deathly fear. Mom called it a phobia. I hated throwing up more than anything in the world. I hated everything about it: the way it looked, the smell, the taste, and that disgusting sound that came with it. Tears squeezed out of my eyes. It would happen any moment.

I would do everything I could to keep myself from getting sick with the flu or food poisoning; it was kind of an obsession. I normally washed my hands about twenty times a day; I breathed inside my shirt when I was around sick people, and I avoided foods that were too spicy or greasy. It worked. Except maybe not this time.

My knees started to ache. I opened my eyes and unplugged my ears while switching to a cross-legged position. I lost count of time.

Different pairs of shoes were going in and out of the stalls next to me. A red pair of high heels clacked into the stall on my left. My legs felt tired again, so I switched back to kneeling. I pulled my face away from the toilet.

Was I feeling better or just imagining it?

I smacked my lips. My mouth wasn't as dry anymore, and I no longer felt like I was going to heave.

Weird.

Getting up from the floor, I heard Ariel's mom: "DJ? Honey?"

"I'm still here," I said as I turned the latch and stepped out of the stall. This was the second or third time she had checked on me.

My name is Dazhoni. You pronounce it Duh-zhoh-nee. Mom and Dad had given my sister and me Navajo names when they were teachers living on a Navajo Indian Reservation. My sister's name is Shundiin, meaning Sunshine, and it's much easier to say than mine. Dazhoni means Beautiful, but I liked to simply go by DJ at my new school.

"The other girls are finishing up shopping," Ariel's mom said as she put her arm around me. "I've been worried. You've been in here almost two hours."

"Two hours?" I repeated. I let her walk me over to a small bench where I rested my head on her shoulder. Mall shopping was over, and the birthday party was over, too.

By the time I was dropped off at home, I felt completely better, even my headache was gone. I was back to my normal self, like being sick had never happened.

"Get some rest," Mom told me after I shared my terrifying and confusing afternoon with her. "At least it's over,"

"Yeah," I agreed, hugging her goodnight.

At least it's over.

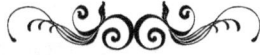

Pull-Ups Competition

"You're not drinking enough water," Mom said when I told her about my headache. She poured me a full glass.

I swallowed a Tylenol capsule and darted to my room to get ready for school. Today was going to be a good day! I didn't usually care for P.E. class, but today we were having a pull-ups competition. Boys were competing against each other and same for the girls.

I wasn't the tallest girl in my class, but I was pretty sure I was the strongest. I did pull-ups on the pipes in our basement all the time, just for fun. I could do as many as twenty. Flinging the closet door open, I thought about wearing my dragon T-shirt today but decided not to. Mom said it looked ridiculous on me because it was way too big. It used to be Dad's, but he gave it to me while he was visiting over winter break. I normally wore it as a night shirt; it was all black with a colorful Chinese dragon on the front.

I loved dragons. They were my favorite animal, even though they were make-believe. They were so cool and strong. I'd be just like one when I won this competition.

I was trying to fit in more at school, so I put on a regular sized hoodie instead. Swinging my backpack over my coat, I followed my sister out the door and into the frigid cold. Mom was already warming up the Jeep.

"I call front seat!" Shundiin shouted through a puff of streaming vapors.

"No!" I shouted back, getting angry. Being older, it should be my right to always ride shotgun. I chased after her pink marshmallow coat heading into the garage. Just as she began to open the passenger door, I rammed into her. "Shun-diiiin!"

"Stop fighting!" Mom scolded and glared at me.

"Yeah, Dazh-oh-neee!" She hopped in and slammed the door shut.

Huffing, I got into the backseat and pressed my throbbing forehead against the frosty window.

My sister was the biggest, most annoying brat in the whole world, and Mom thought she was a perfect princess. We fought all the time and about everything. It hadn't always been like this. We used to like each other before our parents' divorce.

Dad had stayed overseas when we moved back to the States. Life had gotten harder, and Shundiin and I were no longer friends.

"Uh-oh, Dazhoni!" I heard her say while Mom pulled out of the driveway.

"What?" I snarled.

"Quick! Get a bucket – I'm going to throw up!"

"You're just saying that."

"No, really!" She made a gagging noise.

Fear fluttered in my chest. I grabbed the door handle, ready to jump out. "Mom – pull over!" I hollered.

Shundiin giggled. I just wanted to slug her.

"Liar!" I kicked the back of her seat.

"Don't kick!" Of course, Mom only got mad at me.

Once Hawley Elementary came into view, I had to shove aside all my angry thoughts. Inside, Shundiin and I separated down different hallways, hers leading to the third grade classrooms and mine leading to Mr. Lofgren's fifth grade class. I had to tell myself that nothing was going to ruin my day.

After math class, I went to the nurse's office for more Tylenol, but it wasn't helping. Oh, well. I had held down my excitement all morning; P.E. class was next.

At last, it was time for the pull-ups competition! I was so pumped when I lined up behind all the other girls in the gym. And just like I thought, I was the strongest.

I lost count of how many pull-ups I did. I just kept lifting my chin over the bar again and again. Even the boys looked surprised as they watched. I couldn't help but beam at everyone below me. So cool and strong. I could almost feel the fire in my belly and the giant wings sprout from my back.

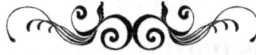

The Doctor Says

Oh no. Oh no.

Those were the words in my head when the doctor said he wanted to check my file. He had asked Mom if I had a history of headaches from allergies or something. When she said no, he typed my information into a computer. He wouldn't find anything about headaches in my history, but he would find out about what a bad kid I was last year. And now I wished I was back at school and that Mom hadn't brought me to Hawley's Clinic.

I used to skip school in fourth grade. I played out an ear infection for as long as I could to stay out of school. I was a bad-tempered trouble maker. Mom tried getting me to talk with a social worker about fighting at home and at school, but I skipped out on that, too.

I didn't know why I did all that stuff. Maybe it was because I only got to see Dad twice a year now. Plus, Mom left her good teaching job overseas to be closer to family. That was hard on Shundiin and me, too.

The doctor had gray, bushy eyebrows, and he raised one of them as he leafed through pages on his clip board and scrolled down his computer. He probably thought I was just trying to skip school again, that the headaches were exaggerated, just like the earaches.

"These headaches have been on and off lately. I've been encouraging her to stay hydrated," Mom said, breaking the silence. "What I don't understand is why Tylenol hasn't been helping; the headaches only seem to eventually go away on their own."

"Hmm." Doctor Shifty Eyebrow gazed directly into my eyes, and I suddenly felt very small. With that look, I knew: he had read bad things about me. I also knew that he didn't take my headaches seriously. He would probably just write me a doctor's note to go back to school tomorrow.

"How's she liking school this year?"

My heart sank. Mom and I were silent.

He stood up and lumbered towards me. Half-heartedly, he went through the motions of feeling my throat and then listening to my heart through his stethoscope.

"If Tylenol doesn't help, she could also try Ibuprofen or Aleve." He then scribbled something on a piece of paper and handed it to Mom. "She can head back to school tomorrow."

I knew it. I knew it.

I hung my head and climbed off the patients' chair. Mom grabbed her purse as I put on my coat. He wasn't going to help. I'd have to wait until the headaches went away on their own.

Mom put her hand on my back once we left the building. "If they continue during the next week or two, I'll make an appointment at the Children's Clinic in Fargo."

I nodded glumly. She was more worried about the headaches than I was. What *I* felt was hurt that the doctor didn't believe me.

A biting wind picked up, and Mom and I hurried to the Jeep as we shielded our faces against the sharp flurries. But could I really blame him? With my history, I wouldn't have believed me either.

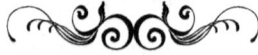

A Basketball Game

"What are Dippin' Dots?"

"They're only the best ice-cream in the world!" Cousin Katie replied in her matter-of-fact voice. She pointed out the small kiosk at the corner of the basketball court, whipping her blond head to the side.

"Mom, can we get some Dippin' Dots? Dazhoni really wants to try them."

"Alright you two, but hurry. The game's about to start."

We stood up as Aunt Vicky forked over a ten-dollar bill. I sheepishly followed my cousin, hopping down the bleachers and weaving through the bystanders. This was how Katie got her mom to buy her stuff. She would say it was my idea and that I wanted them! Aunt Vicky probably thought I was such a demanding niece.

My cousin and I were good friends. She was my favorite part of moving to Hawley. That's why I was disappointed when I found out that she would be in a different fifth grade class than me.

I had sighed with relief when Mom said Cousin Joe's game would end too late for Shundiin to go; the three of us together often got into fights. Mom and Aunt Vicky never believed they started because Shundiin was being a pain. Somehow, it was always my fault or Katie's.

Katie took the second cup from the man at the kiosk and handed it to me. A loud buzzing sound came over the speakers, and I knew the game was about to start. We raced back up the bleachers, pushing past the crowd. As we squished next to Aunt Vicky, the whistle blew and the echoing of the dribbling ball filled the entire gym. It was as if the ball was on loud speakers!

Dippin' Dots were colorful little beads. Yellow, pink, brown and white pieces of ice cream. I let a spoonful melt in my mouth and Katie was right – it *was* the best ice cream in the world!

I searched the gym floor for my lanky high school cousin. Hawley's school colors were maroon and gold; the Detroit Lakes' team was in blue and white.

Someone had already shot a basket and there was cheering and clapping.

Then out of nowhere my stomach did a summersault. My heart began beating louder and louder. *Ba-boom. Ba-boom.* I felt like I was going to be sick! What was happening to me? Did I eat too much junk food today? Was my phobia causing this? I set the Dippin' Dots aside and stared down at the court. I just had to put my mind on something else and the sick feeling would go away.

The hairs began to rise on my neck. I shivered. What if I did throw up? I wondered, feeling scared. Right here in front of all these people. I didn't even know where the bathrooms were in this huge high school. I bunched up my knees and held them to my chest. Getting sick on these bleachers would be the scariest and most embarrassing thing that could ever happen!

I wrapped my coat around me, resting my forehead on my knees. The gym was getting quieter and my heart seemed to be getting louder. I closed my eyes. *Ba-boom. Ba-boom.* Five or six or a million heartbeats rolled by.

I started to hum a song in my mind. It was a new song that we had sung in music class, but for some reason, I couldn't remember the words. At some point I thought I was being poked, but I didn't break my concentration. I thought of a different song. This one named every president, and I had learned it at my last school. When I got to John Quincy Adams for the second time, a magical thing happened: the sick feeling disappeared. It was like poof! The nausea vanished, and my heart was beating normal again.

I opened my eyes and straightened up. A whir of sounds and images blurred together as I tried to refocus on my surroundings. I needed to concentrate on where I was. Soon a whistle blew. More noise. The game was over. Hawley Nuggets had won.

Dazed, I joined Aunt Vicky and Katie in cheering before we stood up to leave. My mind was buzzing with questions. *Why did I get sick? Was it something I ate? The flu? And why am I feeling all better now?*

"Sorry I ate your Dippin' Dots," Katie said with a smile as we left the auditorium. Aunt Vicky rummaged through her purse for her car keys. "But they were melting and you wouldn't wake up."

"That's alright," I told her, not mentioning that I hadn't been sleeping. I had forgotten all about the Dippin' Dots.

Do I tell them what really happened? No. I don't even know what really happened. But it did remind me of Ariel's birthday party.

Katie and I climbed into the back seat. Aunt Vicky started the engine and turned up the heat to full blast. I squinted to read the tiny glow of the car's clock; it was a few minutes after nine. Didn't the game start at seven? And I was sick that whole time. *Almost two hours.*

I stared out the window. On the eerie ride home, I was again reminded of my time in the bathroom stall during Ariel's birthday party at the mall.

Tonight was *exactly* like Ariel's birthday.

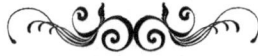

What If?

With my left hand, I chucked the orange prescription bottle against my doorframe. The cap popped off and oval pills littered the carpet of my bedroom. Fuming, I ran down the hall and shoved the front door open. My anger was making my headache worse, but I couldn't hold down my frustration a minute longer.

After more doctor appointments, the headaches still weren't going away; they were getting worse! They hurt even more and would last a whole day or longer. And still nothing helped, not Tylenol, Advil, or Aleve. Or the new migraine pills I was prescribed at my last appointment. The doctor had even told Mom that if the prescription didn't help, that maybe I was just looking for attention, or for an excuse to not go to school. He had suggested that I should see a therapist. I was now missing school as much as I did last year.

By the time I got to our garage, I was on the verge of tears. Clouds hung as heavy and dark as my mood as I strode directly to my lava-colored bike. After five long winter months, I was finally able to grip the handle bars. I charged down the driveway and hopped on. The cool air felt like soft fingers brushing against my throbbing temples.

Riding my bike was my most favorite thing to do in the whole world. I could go anywhere and do anything. I could do wheelies or ride with no hands. I could even go a hundred miles per hour, at least that's what it felt like. I could own the streets of my town. Mom always said I had the balance and agility of a tightrope walker.

Last summer, I had spent most of my days on my bike; I wouldn't have wanted it any other way. On my bike I was free and I was fast. Not being able to ride made my winters depressing.

Down the road I swerved around the stubborn patches of snow that refused to melt. I was sure I looked like a gliding dragon. The wind on my face soothed my pounding headache.

Yesterday Mr. Lofgren had announced that next month our class would be going on an end-of-the-year field trip, along with the other two fifth grade classes. I had almost jumped out of my seat when he said where we were going: Itaska State Park!

Aunt Vicky and Uncle Mike had taken me there last summer. I had had the time of my life pedaling up and down the bike trails with Katie.

The field trip would be several days of camping. I had made sure that Mom signed the permission slip right way. My headaches would be gone by then, for sure; they just had to be. But what if they weren't?

Hitting my break at the end of the road, I suddenly shivered as I turned my bike around to head home. Was it the cold, or was it fear? How long would Mom and I keep running into dead ends with these doctor appointments?

As my block came into view, I thought about my last trip to the clinic. What if the doctor was right? What if the headaches were make-believe? What if they were an excuse to get out of class? I pedaled harder, knowing I was getting upset again.

But if I were making them up, why couldn't I also make them go away? They *had* to be real. Mom believed me, so I had to believe me, too. I parked my bike back inside the garage. My hair was a mess and my head throbbed, but the ride was what I had needed.

Mom and I had to keep going back to the doctors; that was our only plan. The magic medicine was out there somewhere. We just had to find it. And hopefully, before the Itaska field trip.

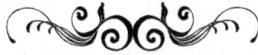

A New Nickname

Itaska was the most spectacular field trip imaginable! There were tons of bike trails with steep hills to race down; there were campfires and the roasting of marshmallows, and there was a river with stepping stones where pictures were taken. Some kids even fell in, but that was part of the fun. Everyone had the greatest time. I could tell from all the happy, laughing faces on the Power Point slideshow that Mr. Lofgren showed the class after the trip was over.

But I wasn't there. Halfway through the slideshow, I bitterly turned away.

My headaches were now lasting all day, every day, with no breaks in between. They were getting worse with each week, even though I thought that wasn't possible. Some days I made it to school, and other days I just gave up on getting out of bed. They never went away.

Could the school year have ended worse? It was the last day of school, and I was dragging my feet out of the nurse's office, again. She was probably tired of seeing me and relieved when Mr. Lofgren called and asked her to send me back to class.

As I turned the corner, a small boy almost ran me over. A lot of kids were breaking the rules and running down the halls today. Everyone was excited that summer vacation was about to start - everyone except me.

"Her reflexes are too brisk," a doctor had told Mom when my headache was so bad that she had taken me to the ER. "She needs an MRI brain scan right away."

Through my tears, I saw Mom's eyes grow as round as moons. *Finally! Someone believes me, and Mom and I are going to get answers!*

But then another doctor had walked in. "She doesn't need an emergency MRI. We could schedule her in for one, but let's try migraine injections first. Our next MRI availability won't be until June Seventeenth, six weeks from now."

I was given a shot and then we headed home. I was almost positive that it wouldn't do any good at all, and I was right. Mom said that maybe it just took time, but I was losing hope that the headaches would ever go away.

As I got to my classroom, I breathed out a defeated sigh and opened the door. Avoiding all the eyes on me, I glanced over to Mr. Lofgren, who gave me a smile and nodded towards my empty desk. I couldn't tell if he believed me about my headaches, but at least he was always nice to me.

All of our desks were now in a circle. At least we weren't going to be watching those Itaska pictures again.

"Now, who's next?" Mr. Lofgren said.

A boy stood up. Blond and with a buzz-cut, Joe always had a crooked grin on his face.

"How about *Corn Dog King*?" the boy sitting next to him suggested.

"Yeah," someone else chimed in. "No one's as happy as Joe when corn dogs are on the menu!"

Chuckles erupted across the room.

And no one is spared from his bragging about how many he could eat. I kept my thoughts to myself.

"Yep, that's me!" Joe quipped as he sat back down.

A girl sitting next to him stood up. She was on the basketball team and was always the first to be picked when the class split into teams during P.E. She always wore her black, frizzy hair in a pony tail, out of her way. Several kids offered suggestions for her nickname, but I wasn't paying attention any longer. Twirling a pencil under my empty desk, I wondered what nickname my classmates would give me. No one knew me very well. But maybe, *Lefty*? Mr. Lofgren had once mentioned that there were only two of us lefties in the entire class.

My turn. When I got to my feet, I heard sharp whispers around the circle before it grew quiet. I had told Mom about the whispering some of the girls did when I had returned from the nurse's office one day. I was certain they were making fun of me, but Mom assured me that I was just being over sensitive.

"How about *Miss Never Here*?" a girl with freckles volunteered. "Everyone knows she hides out in the nurse's office so she doesn't have to be in class."

There was snickering across the room as Mr. Lofgren cast her a disapproving look. My face grew really hot.

Mr. Lofgren quickly began talking about what a smart, creative girl I was. He gave me a different nickname, but I was too embarrassed to pay attention. When I sat back down, I sunk deep into my seat, wishing the floor could turn to quicksand and swallow me up.

At least I won't be seeing anyone here for a while, I thought. Everything in our house was now in boxes. Mom, Shundiin, and I would be moving back to the Rothsay home for the summer, maybe longer. We would head back next week, right around the time our report cards arrived in the mail.

Katie had told me that I was lucky to have passed after missing over forty days of school. I couldn't wait to be out of here.

Our class made it through the rest of the circle right before the bell rang. Suddenly it was like fireworks had gone off. Mr. Lofgren cheerfully dismissed us, and I squeezed past the excited frenzy of kids on my way to my locker. Summer vacation was now here, and there was still no cure for my headaches. At that moment, I couldn't tell if my head hurt more or my heart.

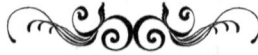

The Magic Pill

"Welcome to Burger King, may I take your order?"

"We'll have two Whopper Juniors and - " AJ's mom stuck her head back inside the car window. "What would you like, Sweetie?"

I wasn't hungry, but she insisted that I eat something. "Um, a salad," I said, aware of how weak my voice sounded.

"And we'll take a salad. Thank you." AJ's mom said before pulling up to the pay window.

"A *salad*?" AJ raised her eyebrows.

I tried to smile but was sure it was more like a wince. "I like salad," I said. That was a big fat lie and my best friend knew it.

I hadn't eaten since yesterday afternoon when I first arrived for the sleepover, and AJ's mom thought that was the reason I felt so sick.

This morning I had just gotten over one of my nauseous episodes, and I was scared to eat. I chose a salad because I figured I could move the pieces of lettuce around to make it look like I was eating. Easier to fake than pretending to eat a hamburger.

At the second window, AJ's mom handed back a Whopper Junior and the salad. The late morning sunlight glistened through AJ's dirty blond hair as she unwrapped her burger. The smell of mayonnaise and tomatoes filled the backseat while she took a bite in silence. She wasn't her usual hyper and talkative self, and that was because of me. I had ruined the birthday of another friend.

Last night my headache was so bad that I thought my head was going to burst open. It had been as painful as the time when mom had taken me to the ER. What a rotten night. We had pitched up a tent in her front yard, and AJ had brought some board games from her dad's house. Even though I hadn't finished unpacking from our move back to Rothsay, I was able to find my soccer ball. Bad idea. Running around had made my headache even worse.

I hadn't slept at all; I ended up crying and writhing about in my sleeping bag all night. AJ woke up several times and crept into her house to get me

Ibuprofen, which of course, didn't help. At day-break I was nothing but nauseous. I felt relieved to be finally going home. If the sleepover had been at AJ's dad's, I could've gone home anytime, since he was our next-door neighbor.

I picked at the salad and then set it down. Trying not to think, I wrapped my arms around my head and listened to the humming of the car engine. My thoughts grew dark. How much longer could I live like this? How much longer until my head actually did explode? And how much longer until I could have fun and be myself again? I didn't expect those questions to be answered anytime soon.

⁓⚬⚬⚬⚬⁓

The ice pack was gently lifted from my face. My tears blurred the image of Mom as she sat down at the corner of my bare bed; my sheets were still in a suitcase somewhere. I rubbed my eyes. She was holding a glass of water and two pills. "Your dad wanted me to tell you that he understood why you couldn't talk to him on the phone, so don't feel bad about it. I told him everything. He said he wanted you to try these – they're Excedrin. He said that he took these whenever he got headaches."

I sat up. I must've given her a look.

"I know, nothing has worked. But let's just give them a try."

If my head didn't hurt so bad, I would've rolled my eyes. Noticing the 'E' engraved on them, I picked the pills out of her hand and swallowed them, then laid back down to settle into my self-pity thoughts.

It couldn't have been very long, though. Maybe thirty minutes.

Presto!

I dug my small stereo out of a box and searched for a radio station with the loudest song. Leaping back onto my bed, I furiously strummed my air guitar. I began jumping up and down. My world had just changed! The pain was gone, and I was back to feeling like me again. Dad had found it – the magic pill. It was the miracle I'd been waiting for.

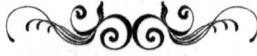

Cloud Nine

SWOOSH!

At the bottom of the hill, I slammed on my brake and came to a stop. My jeans were soaked. Gliding over to the side of the road, I could hear Cody speeding down the hill towards the puddle. Last time around I hadn't moved out of the way and I had gotten soaked.

I brushed my dripping hair out of my face. No headaches for a week, and bike riding all day. I felt like I was on top of the world.

I shielded my eyes as Cody reached the puddle with a *SWOOSH!* and a shout. His pants were as soaked as mine.

Cody was a friend I had from Mrs. Krueger's fourth grade class here in Rothsay. He didn't actually live in town, but his grandma did. While cruising around, I had found him riding his bike, too. That led to showing him the huge puddle left from last night's storm.

Since the discovery of Excedrin, it was like I was high up in the clouds and there was no coming down! I kept the bottle of pills in my room, taking two at a time every four hours to keep the headaches at bay. I didn't tell Mom that I took the maximum dose allowed – eight pills in twenty-four hours. By the time the pain started coming back, I knew it was time to take the next dose. I felt that I had turned into the Energizer Bunny, eager to make up for all the fun times the headaches had taken away. The caffeine ingredient probably made me a bit too jumpy.

Cody turned his bike around, getting ready to pedal up the hill again. I stared out into the street and wondered what time it was. I could see our Jeep parked in front of our house not far away.

I was kind of frustrated with Mom for making me go to the scheduled MRI appointment in Fargo today. It was cutting into the time I could spend on my bike. I was almost all better now, no thanks to any of those doctors. I had the magic pills, and all that was left for me to do now was to keep taking them until it made my headaches go away for good. I had begged Mom to cancel the MRI and let me stay home, but she didn't give in.

I turned to Cody. "Hey, I'm gonna head back home now. I've got to change and go to Fargo with my mom."

"Oh, okay." he replied a bit sullenly. "I'll be back at my grandma's next weekend. Will I see you then?"

"Definitely!"

I pedaled off hoping the puddle would still be there next week. I would get this last doctor's appointment out of the way and then concentrate on the good times up ahead. Holding my chin high, I stopped peddling and let the wind make ripples through my T-shirt as I daydreamed about my summer.

After another few weeks of bike riding and tree-climbing, Dad would be coming in early July. Being with him was always a highlight. During summer and Christmas vacations, he stayed at a hotel with a swimming pool and made it the best time for Shundiin and me. Last year, he had also rented a cabin at a lake resort, and he said we would do it again this summer. Rain or shine, nothing would stop me from swimming all day.

Dad had even bought fishing poles for us last time. Impaling the worms with hooks and then taking the fish off them was too gross for us, so Dad took care of that part. Three weeks with Dad! The only hard thing would be saying good-bye again when he flew back to China.

But then there was August, the month of my birthday. What would my birthday be like this year? Could I convince Mom to let me invite a bunch of my friends over, like Ariel, AJ, Cody, and Katie for a water-balloon fight? That would be awesome!

Coasting up to my front yard, I set my bike down on the freshly mown lawn and glanced back across the empty street, at the puddle. I promised myself I would be over there again later this afternoon.

I certainly wasn't going to let this time-wasting doctor appointment stop me. The corners of my mouth stretched to hug my face. I wasn't going to take my headache-free summer for granted; I would make the best memories ever, and it was going to be the most amazing summer of my life.

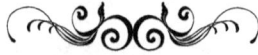

A Brain Tumor

"Let's name your brain tumor Jimmy."

Katie was standing behind me at the bottom of the stairs; she reached up a lanky arm and rapped her knuckles on the side of my head. "Helloo, Jimmy!"

We burst out laughing.

We began to head upstairs to my room when Aunt Vicky called out, "Hot dogs are ready!" Katie and I immediately spun around and headed out the back door.

"Two, please!" I was so hungry! I grabbed a paper plate and held it up to my aunt as she stood over the sizzling grill. After she plunked two scorched and blistered hotdogs onto my plate, I plastered them with ketchup. Katie did the same. We sat next to each other at the picnic table; Shundiin and her friend, Marissa, sat across from us, already eating.

Aunt Vicky had brought Marissa with her from Hawley so that Shundiin had someone to play with, too. She and Mom had to talk about the MRI results and the plans for my emergency surgery up ahead. My MRI showed that I had a *mass* in my brain: a tumor.

"What's a tumor?" I had asked Mom when we were leaving the doctor's office. She had tried to explain. I imagined something like a chicken nugget stuck inside my head. It was the cause of my head-aches and my spells of nausea.

"Guess what?" I turned around to face the grown-ups. "We named my brain tumor Jimmy!" While Katie and I went into another round of giggles, Mom and Aunt Vicky didn't even smile.

They were in a sullen mood, and Mom had this grave expression that hadn't left her face since our doctor appointment. But the image on the scan was the proof I had needed to show everyone that the headaches were real. I wasn't crazy, and I wasn't making them up, either! All we had to do now was get the tumor out so that the headaches would be gone for good, and I could stop taking Excedrin. Why were the adults so glum?

"How about you girls go to the park and play?" Mom finally replied, giving me a look that said this wasn't just a suggestion.

I nodded, knowing she and Aunt Vicky wanted some alone time. I shoved the end of my second hot-dog into my mouth and washed it down with some cherry Kool-Aid.

"Come on, guys!" I grabbed my bike and mounted up. I would be the only one on a bike, but that wasn't my problem. The other girls would just have to try to keep up with me! Like a rocket, I blasted off towards East Park. Taking my hands off the handlebars, I sat up straight and did my balancing act.

"Show off!" my sister shouted. Realizing I was a little too far ahead of them, I slowed down so that Mom wouldn't yell at me.

"Wow! So you're going to Mayo Clinic?" My friend Emily had stared at me wide-eyed earlier today, when I had ridden over to the tiny business building called Partners where her mom worked. I had told them about the headaches and about going to Mayo Clinic. "You'll like it there. It's ginormous!" Emily had said. "It has all these sculptures and paintings inside, just like a museum."

I didn't tell her that I thought museums were boring. But I had reminded myself that being bored and getting stitches would be worth it to be rid of my headaches and nausea.

I had thought getting the scan would be the last of seeing doctors, but the MRI actually made me need more appointments. It turned this week into a busy one. Tomorrow, Mom, Shundiin, and I would make the three-hour trip to Buffalo, Minnesota, and we'd spend the night at Aunt Sandy's and Uncle Dennis' house. Then another two-hour drive to Rochester for an appointment with the surgeon. The following morning would be my surgery. And hopefully, no more doctors and appointments for the rest of my summer.

The sound of footsteps told me that the others were right behind me.

I had never had stitches before. But when I was in first grade, a boy in my class fell on some ice and busted his lip open. When he came back the next day, he had stitches sewn on his chin. I imagined it would be like that, but with the stitches somewhere on my head. I wondered why the doctors couldn't just use tweezers and pull the tumor out from my ear.

The park came into view up ahead, and the sun was starting to set. The sky had become a tinted pastel orange and pink. I put away my thoughts of surgery. The other girls were already chasing toward the jungle gym. Before dropping my bike near the swings, I pulled up on my handlebars to do one more wheelie. Unknown to me then, it would be my very last wheelie ever.

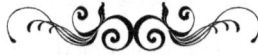

Goodbye Jimmy

My finger traced the black mythical creature on my shorts – its long, jagged body and its spear-like tail. A majestic dragon.

Mom and I were sitting on cushy chairs in the lobby of St. Mary's Hospital. It was early, the earliest appointment that I had ever had. I wasn't allowed to eat or drink anything since midnight, and no Excedrin, even though I had a full-blown headache.

Today was the big day. The day Jimmy would be out of my head. The day my life would go back to normal, and the last of my headaches. The moment I had woken up this morning, I had decided to wear my new, favorite shorts. I had spotted them in the boys' swimsuit isle during our trip to Walmart the day before. One side of the shorts was red, and the other side was white, but it was the sleek, black dragon down the right side that had prompted me to beg Mom for them. Even though Mom had told me that I would be asleep during the operation, I wanted to be wearing my cool shorts when I woke up, when I was healthy and pain-free, strong like the dragon.

In hardly no time, a nurse in scrubs met us in the lobby and brought me to a changing room. She handed me an ugly gown and shower cap. I slumped my shoulders when she told me I couldn't wear my cool shorts; this wasn't starting out the way I had planned.

I'll just have to change into my shorts as soon as my surgery is done, I told myself when I stepped out from the curtain. A long table on wheels was waiting for me, along with another nurse in scrubs. I laid on my back and was pushed down one hall and then another. A right turn, then a left; it was kind of fun except for my head pounding to the rhythm of the nurses' quick steps. *BOOM. BOOM. BOOM.*

I started to think about the appointment I had had with Dr. Raffel yesterday. When Mom and I had left his office, I was really upset.

The appointment was at two o'clock, but Dr. Raffel had an emergency surgery and was running very late. The Excedrin I had taken before Mom and I left the Comfort Inn had worn off, and I hadn't brought any extra. I was also hungry. Finally, Mom and I were led into Dr. Raffel's office; the neurosurgeon had pulled up the images of my brain scan, and he discussed my surgery with Mom. He had used many words and terms that I didn't know, but I did understand some of it. *Eight weeks . . . balance and coordination.* I wasn't paying close attention until he said *nausea center.*

"Removing the tumor in the cerebellum will also affect this area along the brain stem, right here, the area postrema – it's the nausea center of the brain." He circled the spot on the screen with his finger. "She will become very ill."

What? Wasn't the surgery supposed to make me all better? Did he mean that I was going to throw up? A volcano of fear had erupted inside of me. When the appointment was over, I had barely noticed as Mom led us out to the lobby.

I've made it all these months without throwing up during my nausea spells. What if it finally happens tomorrow after surgery? What if I don't just throw up once, but throw up all day long? What if another day of my summer is lost?

I couldn't help it; I cried.

Mom had called her friend who had volunteered to watch Shundiin at the hotel. "The doctor was running late because of an emergency surgery, but Dazhoni and I are heading back now. Hm? The Ronald McDonald House called back about an availability? That's great! Yes, we'll spend the night there instead."

I had leaned into Mom, my tears making everything a blur. "I don't want to throw up after surgery! Why will I throw up?" If the surgery was going to make me vomit, I didn't want to have it!

Now, here I was staring up at the ceiling . . . *the Big Day*. I was pushed into a room where I spotted a familiar face. "Mom!" She was sitting there waiting for me. In another corner of the room were other people, also lying on rolling beds and wearing shower caps.

When my nurse walked away for a moment, I pointed at my head. "Do I look like a washy woman?" I giggled. Mom smiled and put her hand on my face. I hoped being silly would calm both of us. I decided that since I had followed Dr. Raffel's instructions of not eating or drinking anything since last night, I wouldn't throw up. I just *had* to be all better after surgery.

The nurse returned and Mom kissed me, telling me she'd see me when I woke up. My rolling bed was then pushed through two large swinging doors, into a room where everything was a glaring white. The walls, the floor, the ceiling. I hardly recognized Dr. Raffel as he stood next to another man; he wore a mask like the kind dentists wear, and also a shower cap. Funny thing, he also wore shower caps on his shoes. This was the cleanest, most sterile looking room I had ever seen. All I could smell was hand sanitizer.

This was it. My chest got fluttery. I clutched the gown at my sides, wishing I was wearing my dragon shorts. When I came out of this room there would be no more Excedrin, and no more headaches. But first, I had to go to sleep. How were they going to make me do that?

"What flavor would you like?" asked a man dressed just like Dr. Raffel. "Grape, cherry, cotton candy, or bubble gum?"

"Bubble gum," I answered, wondering why he asked me that. A plastic mask with a hose was then attached to my face, and I could taste a light mist coming out of it. *Mmm. Bubble gum.*

I took a breath. Even if I did throw up afterwards, I told myself, I would soon be better. I just had to be brave. Feeling my eyelids sag, my fingers let go of my gown. After today, I would be myself again. Riding my bike, playing at the park, swimming with Dad; all without having to take my magic pills.

I took another breath.

After today, I'll be as strong as a dragon.

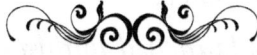

Real Life?

It was the scariest, most horrible nightmare I ever had. I was in some kind of twirling, upside down universe that wouldn't stop spinning. Around, around, around. Sickening.

Everything was wrong. Gravity was completely off, I couldn't stop falling; down, down. Although I was lying flat on a gurney, even the tongue in my mouth felt like it was falling.

So nauseous.

I was hurting so badly, but I couldn't tell where the pain was coming from. The back of my head and nape felt damp and stiff.

Every kind of pain and nausea that I had ever known before was now a joke. A hideous joke.

I couldn't even bring myself to open my eyes. I knew this place would be terrifying.

Time passed. Was it a minute or a million minutes? There was no way to know.

There were voices; muffled sounds like I was listening from under a heavy, gooey muck. I lifted my chin just a little, but I shouldn't have.

It felt like I was launched within a runaway elevator that suddenly stopped. My stomach lurched. Any movement I made shook the ground and swept me into a whirlpool of dizziness. Trapped, I had to keep perfectly still.

More than anything, I wanted to wake up. I waited for the moment my dream legs would rescue me, kick me out of the depths of this horror land and into the real and normal world up on the surface. I waited, but that moment never came. Hours wore out and fell away.

⚜

"Hey, kiddo, it's Dr. Raffel. Can you wiggle your toes for me?

Good. I'm placing my finger in the palm of your hand. Can you squeeze? Very good."

Eyes opened.

Inside Horror Land.

Walls. Ceilings. Moving. Colliding.

SOUVENIRS OF SUFFERING

Mom's voice.

Turning.

Earthquake.

Vomitting. Shaking.

Please . No more.

Urp!. More vomit.

Face wiped. Propped up. Held tight.

Clean gown.

A nurse. Blue scrubs.

Two heads. Four eyes.

Closing my eyes.

I need to wake up!

꧁⁂꧂

51

There was a knocking on the door.

"How is she?"

"Dr. Raffel." Mom's voice. "She's in and out. She was awake a little while ago. But she's been vomiting and she's unable to hold herself up. This isn't from the anesthesia, is it?"

"It's due to the location of where the tumor had been. What she's feeling right now is similar to what a severely intoxicated person would feel: nausea, loss of balance, and double vision. Pretty much what I had described during our initial appointment. But like I said, she should be feeling better after about eight weeks."

So. There will be no waking up from HorrorLand. This is real life. How could the surgery have gone so wrong? Yet Dr. Raffel isn't surprised by what the operation has done to me. It's me that is so wrong. This is my reality.

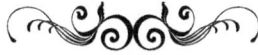

Helpless

A swirl of colors. Rolling down a hallway. Moving shapes. Square tiles. Swimming. Drowning. I was sitting in a wheel chair that turned around, then headed back towards my room.

"You're doing such a great job taking care of your big sister." Mom's voice. "The nurse thinks it would be a good idea to give her a shower, but we have to keep the back of her head dry. The nurse and I are going to lift her into the chair, so if you could grab those towels for me."

"Okay, Mom." Shundiin's voice.

My gown was taken off and my eyepatch removed. My double vision was back. I tried to lift myself up, but hands gripped me tightly.

"Don't try to move about on your own - we don't want another situation like this morning," Mom said to me. I kept forgetting that I had no balance, that this was my new body. I stared down at my bare thighs. If I moved my head just slightly, I knew I would vomit.

I heard the faucet turn. Cold water sprayed across my knees. I shuddered. "Uhh." Even my mouth seemed to have no balance. My words wouldn't come out right.

"Oh! Sorry, honey. Was that too cold?" Again, I heard the faucet being turned.

I wanted to feel the back of my head, but something was wrong with my arms, especially my left one. I tried to lift it again, but it just flopped about on its own. Which way was up and which way was down? I couldn't tell anymore. My fingers finally found it. A thick, bumpy strip down to the nape of my neck. This was my new head.

"Make sure all the soap is rinsed off." Mom's voice. The faucet shut off and I was dried with a towel.

Mom, Shundiin and the nurse were seeing me naked. I wanted to feel embarrassed, but I couldn't. I also wanted to feel scared and mad and sad, but I couldn't feel that either. I couldn't feel anything except pain and nausea and dizziness. I couldn't *feel* my feelings anymore.

"Nurse? Do you know why my daughter seems so - I don't know . . . stoic?" Mom's voice again.

Once more fitted into a gown, I was team lifted onto my bed.

"She has what we call *flat affect*. It can result from traumatic brain injuries and surgeries. She's in a state of shock."

A whirring sound came from the bed, and I was lying down once again. I closed my eyes. An emotionless zombie. This was the new me.

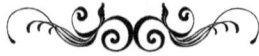

Occupational Therapy

Not these, I thought, clutching the brim of the sink with all my might. My legs trembled as the occupational therapist pulled the shorts up to my waist. She hadn't put my eye patch on yet, so everything I looked at had a duplicate shadow.

Simply looking at my new world made me feel sick. I kept my eyes shut. My knees buckled, and I let myself fall into the wheelchair propped behind me. The therapist grumbled something and turned on the faucet. She was a sturdy woman with a deep, gruff voice.

I hated that she had me up at seven every miserable morning, helped me into a wheelchair, helped me use the toilet, get dressed, and then wash my face and brush my hair. Keeping my head down, I stared into my lap. Red and white. The black dragon on my right. I had almost forgotten I had these shorts; they were a dream from another world.

Something warm and damp dropped into my hand. A crumpled washcloth. It took my clumsy fingers forever to open and grip it; to lift it up and find my face. My hands refused to do what my brain was telling them. With an awkward swiping motion, the cloth brushed across my cheeks, then I felt it being taken away. I decided it was good that I couldn't feel my feelings; I would be embarrassed at how klutzy I was. Keeping my head as still as possible to avoid another earthquake, I continued to stare at the shorts. Why had Mom given me these to wear? Why my *cool* shorts?

A small hairbrush was placed into my right hand. The therapist instructed me to look in the mirror while I brushed my hair. She obviously had no idea of what I went through every time I lifted my head. All of my muscles tensed and I clenched my teeth as I lifted my chin.

I waited for the spinning tornado to stop. And when it did, my gaze was set straight above the sink. Two pairs of glassy, vacant eyes were looking back at me. Two diagonal mouths, slightly open, drooling, pasted to an emotionless face, a face that had a second one shadowed beneath it. This was the first time I saw myself after surgery, and it didn't seem like me at all. This was an opposite of the independent girl who could do wheelies, run fast, wrinkle her nose and roll her eyes at her sister.

That girl was now gone. The only thing left of her were the thoughts in my head right now. I forgot about the hairbrush in my hand until I heard it drop to the floor.

Who was I looking at in the mirror? If I couldn't do all the things I used to do, was I still me?

Who am I?

I slowly lowered my head and stared into my lap as the therapist took over brushing my hair. Dully staring at the black dragon on my shorts, I had another thought: *I don't deserve to wear these. I'm not cool anymore.*

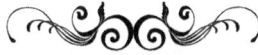

Physical Therapy

Step.

A swirl of sounds and movements surrounded me. I kept my head as low and still as I could. *Come on.* I concentrated.

Step.

My physical therapist cheered me on. "Keep going, you're halfway there!"

She seemed to be clapping from miles away, where the two metal bars ended. I only wanted to finish this so I could lie back down. Even when I was still, I was engulfed in a dizziness that made it impossible to tell which way was up, down, left or right. I relied on my trembling arms to tell me what direction I was going. Reach and pull. Reach. Pull. Forward.

Dad would be here any day now. Each night of my new life I was hoping that tomorrow would be the day I'd feel better, just in time for him to see me. Tomorrow would be the day I'd wake up as myself. I would forget that all this had happened, and I would still have an awesome summer with Dad. And I didn't want him to come until that day; I didn't want him to see me like this.

Step.

Too fast. My head swayed to the side.

Dizziness.

My stomach launched into my throat.

Nauseous.

I held on tighter.

Keep going. A voice echoed in my ears.

Another step.

Another. I made it.

"That was awesome, girl! Good job!" My physical therapist had told me that yesterday, too, even though I hadn't made it to the end of the bars. As my legs began to give out, she supported me, then turned me about so I could sink back into the wheelchair.

"You must be tired," she said in that same drawn-out way.

"Yeah …" I flatly replied as she pushed me through the large, white doors.

Almost all of the therapists and nurses talked to me that way now. They raised the volume of their voices and pronounced each word extra clearly, as if I couldn't hear well, or like I was having a hard time understanding them. But I could hear and understand them just fine. Although I knew I must look like a zombie, I wished they could just talk to me normally.

We turned a corner and I recognized the colorful wall tiles. We were back in the pediatrics unit. Almost to my room. I heard voices near my door and imagined that Mom was talking to the aide who brought my meals. I didn't smell the food yet, but I knew what would happen once I did. I vomited every time I caught a whiff of the food cart once it entered my room.

I wanted to tell the physical therapist to turn around and go back, but the only sound that came out of me was a soft groan. I prepared myself as the therapist pushed me inside. I knew I was going to get sick all over my lap.

With my eyes focused on the floor, I realized there was no smell of food. Instead, I was looking at some large, man-sized tennis shoes; they were attached to blue jeans and they were striding towards me. I knew exactly who it was, and more than anything I wanted to feel some emotion. I lifted my head. So dizzy...

I was looking at a swirl of colors. A blurry oval. Then a face with teary eyes. Dad.

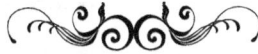

Malignant

Mom had said that she and Dad had to talk to me about something serious. From the tone of her voice, I could tell it was something bad. *The talk* would happen once Dad and I were back from our walk.

Dad held out his arm, making an L-shape by bending his elbow. I placed my arm over his and gripped his hand as he pulled me up, out of the wheelchair. With our arms locked together, he supported some of my weight and held me securely as I staggered alongside him. With his help, I didn't need someone on each side of me. This was how we took our walks.

Two, sometimes three times a day, Dad wheeled me out here to St. Mary's courtyard. We left the wheelchair behind and walked around the fountain, stopping at each bench along the way. Sunlight dappled the walkway and our shadows followed, then led the way around the path. Dr. Raffel had told my parents that I needed to walk as often as I could, and Dad had taken it upon himself to see that I did.

"Years ago, I cut my hand while working on an art project. I had to get stitches and my hand didn't work like it used to. But I kept using it to draw and paint. Now, it works just fine." He showed me the scars across his fingers. "What happened to me is minor compared to what you're going through, but I know the neurologist is right - the more you walk, the better your balance will get."

Like Mom and Shundiin, Dad didn't talk to me slowly or loudly, even though I no longer had a personality and only said a word or two at a time. I felt alright with him seeing me like this; he knew that deep inside I was still the same me.

Always positive and encouraging, Dad did most of the talking on our walks. But this afternoon he didn't say much. I knew he was thinking about the talk he and Mom were going to have with me.

"Would you like to walk around the fountain one more time?" he asked when we got to the last bench.

"No..." With my head down, I lifted my shaky arm to point to where I thought the doors of the hospital were. After my wobbly legs felt rested, I wanted to muster the strength to walk to my wheel-chair so that we could get back and have our *talk*.

I knew it would be about my condition. They'd start off by saying, *You're very sick, sicker than you had expected*. But was there anything else left to say? I knew now how foolish I'd been to have joked about my tumor; it wasn't anything to laugh about. I hadn't understood the seriousness of it then, but I did now.

Was I in trouble for giving my brain tumor a silly name and turning it into a joke? Because I was sorry now; I would never do that again.

Lying back in bed, I quickly realized that I wasn't in trouble. Mom and Dad held my hands and I could sense they were struggling with what they had to tell me. Finally, Mom said I was still very ill, and that the doctors had discovered that my tumor was *malignant*. Even if I guessed all night, I wouldn't have been able to figure out what that meant.

Dad then told me that I had a very serious dis-ease. His voice seemed weighted with worry, though he smiled down at me encouragingly. I had heard of people dying from this disease; and I had thought it was something that only old people got, not a kid.

I had cancer.

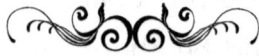

Reality Check

"We're home!" I cried exuberantly.

From the passenger window of Dad's silver rental car I could see my bike lying where I had left it in our front yard. Shadows timidly huddled on the porch steps, hiding from the soft afternoon sunlight.

It felt amazing to be back! I swiped the eye patch off my face and stepped outside. The nausea and dizziness were gone. My coordination and balance were back to normal.

Today was July 9th, the day the doctors had told me I could go home, so here I was, all better now. All the pain and sickness had melted off during the long drive back to Rothsay, hundreds of miles away from St. Mary's Hospital. Far away from my surgery and everything it had done to me.

My heart fluttered as I made a running leap up the front steps to the crooked screen door. I was back. Back to my old world, the one that made sense. Back to the real me. The active, independent, ready-for-fun, healthy me . . .

"Careful, honey."

The sound of plastic bouncing off the pavement brought me out of my daydream. I dully gazed at my legs dangling outside the passenger door of Dad's rental car; I had accidentally kicked out the green bowl that Dad had brought along for me to throw up in. Vertigo swam over me.

Dad set the bowl back under my seat and unbuckled my seatbelt. We locked arms and I ducked my head like I had practiced with the simulated car door in physical therapy. With a swoop, Dad hoisted me up to my feet. We had only been on the road home for a short time when Dad had decided it would be a good idea to grab something to eat.

My legs began to shake after only a few moments of waiting for Mom and Shundiin to park the Jeep and join us. I was still hoping, still waiting for the magical moment when I'd feel all better; because today was the day the doctors had told me I could go home.

Dad gripped my arm tightly as we stepped inside Subway. Was this the same Subway where Mom, Shundiin and I had stopped on our trip down to Rochester, just a couple weeks ago? The one in the normal world where Shundiin and I had made our own special drinks, mixing all the flavors together from the soda machine? Yep. And it was just as crowded. But now, all of the sounds and smells were overwhelming. It was too much, like it was suffocating me. Voices came from every direction of the room. The strong smell of deli meats and bread made me feel more nauseas.

Shundiin scouted out for an open table, and Mom pulled out one of the chairs for me. I willed my body to stay upright and struggled to keep my head up while the three of them queued in line to order.

Families were scattered about at different tables; couples were talking, kids were laughing. Everything was so normal for them; their world hadn't been pulled out from beneath their feet over the past two weeks. It didn't feel right. I didn't belong in the same world that they were in, not while I was like this. I huddled into myself, willing myself to become smaller and smaller, hoping no one would notice me.

Mom returned with napkins and drinks, and Dad had a tray of sandwiches. I had told him that I wasn't hungry, but he brought me back a six-inch turkey sub anyway. Shundiin had grabbed a lid and straw for my cup of water.

Now for the hard part – picking up the cup of water steadily and carefully. I had spent many mornings in physical therapy with plastic pegs in front of me, and it had taken all my powers of concentration to focus enough to grasp them with my fumbling fingers and insert them into the holes in the block of foam. It was like my hands and fingers had forgotten how to do the simplest things. Using my right hand, which was less shaky, I concentrated on holding the paper cup and lifting it towards me.

As I reached out, my entire arm disappeared from my field of vision. When it reappeared, my hand swiped against the cup. *Okay. Now grab slowly.* The cup was shaking. *Lift,* I told myself. I felt the weight of the cup as I lifted it closer. *Closer.* The straw jabbed against my forehead, and I instinctively jerked my arm back. Yet somehow, my hand and cup were going in the opposite direction.

A soft cry escaped my throat as I felt cold water and ice pour down my back. I blinked in surprise, but was unable to feel any other emotion as the empty cup was gently taken from my hand.

Mom and Dad jumped up right away as they grabbed wads of napkins. Their metal chairs screeched against the linoleum floor, breaking the silence.

I just then noticed how quiet and still the noisy Subway had become. Shivering, I realized my back was soaked. Shundiin was cleaning up the spill near my feet, and Mom and Dad were wiping off my shoulder and back.

Everyone is looking at me. Probably wondering why this stupid girl dumped her drink over her shoulder like that. I don't belong in the normal world anymore. I don't want to go home today. Not like this.

During the rest of the drive home, all of my hopes of being back to my old self faded away with every mile. By the time I finally wobbled and swayed through the front door of our home, there was nothing left but disappointment.

We were home, but I wasn't back.

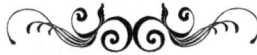

Don't Stare At Me

Hurry!

With my hands bracing each side of the door frame, I felt my knees begin to buckle. Dad finished tying my shoe just in time to hold up some of my weight. We were now arm in arm.

I breathed a heavy sigh, reminded of when Dad had brought me with him to Kmart a few days ago. *Hurry*, I had said to myself when he had let go of me for a moment to grab something off the shelf. I had clutched the cart's handle bar with both hands, fearful that my legs would give out. But Dad had locked his arm back into mine just in time.

"Ready?" he asked, reaching for my eyepatch. He straightened it under my glasses.

"Ready," I replied in my monotone voice as we cautiously headed down the front steps.

Actually, I never felt ready to leave my green puking bowl behind when we left for our walks. What if I needed it? But Dad had said if we waited until I didn't feel nauseous, I wouldn't be leaving my bed for ages! He was determined to keep us regimented with our walks ever since returning from the hospital. I just hoped I wouldn't get sick while we were out.

We took the same fifteen-minute walk each time – a circle around the block. The sun beamed down on us as we turned the first corner by the old church, making slow progress with wobbly steps. If I didn't have Dad's arm locked onto mine, I would probably be sitting on the sidewalk. I had to concentrate on each step before I took it. *Right leg forward. Left leg forward. Right. Left.*

Whenever I lost concentration, my brain would forget which leg was already forward and I'd nearly trip. Good thing Dad always sensed when this happened and he would hold me securely.

Both Mom and Dad were with me all the time now. While we were still at the hospital in Rochester, Aunt Vicky had fixed up our family's guest bedroom as my new room. It was downstairs and it had its own bathroom. Aunt Vicky had also bought me a new bed with *Finding Nemo* bedsheets and pillowcases. My whole family had moved downstairs to be closer to me; Shundiin was in the former office room, and Mom and Dad slept on couches in the living room and family room.

I had started vomiting this morning before it was light. I had been afraid to climb out of bed because I didn't want to fall in the dark. Luckily, Dad had heard me. Within seconds he had rushed in and turned on the light. He dumped out my bowl and then rubbed my back.

Mom and Dad were getting along better than they ever had since their divorce; and if I could have felt my feelings, I would've been so happy about that.

We turned the next corner and passed a small house. Their yard was filled with brightly colored gnomes and other decorations, and off to the side, I could see two elderly people sitting in lawn chairs. I could feel them staring in our direction.

"Good afternoon," Dad greeted.

Dizziness clouded about me as I lifted my head to smile, but as I looked at them, they quickly glanced away. I waited for them to look back in my direction, but they wouldn't.

I dropped my head back down as we passed their home. *Why'd they do that?* Maybe their parents had taught them that it was rude to stare at people who were different, but I wished they could see past my condition and just smile back at me. We turned another left, and I could feel my legs getting weaker.

"Almost back," Dad encouraged as I shifted more of my weight onto him. We were past the half way mark. I lifted my eyes to the quiet street. A month ago, I was zooming across here on my bike. So fast and graceful, cutting sharp corners all around – like a cheetah. Up ahead, I spotted our neighbor's beige house. AJ's teenage brother was standing next to their clothesline, his blond hair appearing white from the sun's glare. He was facing our way, eyes glued on something.

"Oo-ooh, you have a crush on my big brother!" AJ used to tease me.

"Do not!" I had insisted. At least I hadn't thought I had. I just thought he was super cool. When I had gotten my new Gameboy Advance games, I had shown him how advanced I was, in an attempt to impress him. I had wanted him to think I was pretty cool, too. Now look at me, I thought. Instead of a cheetah, I move like a drunken robot. To make things worse, as we got closer, I realized he was staring in my direction, staring at me.

I had a sudden urge to hide behind Dad. Even though I had wished that the old couple had taken a second to meet my eyes, at least they hadn't been gawking at me. *Stop it, Devin! Don't you know it's not polite to stare?*

His eyes burned holes through me, and I just kept walking past with my head down, waiting for it to be over. It was the first time I felt an emotion since my surgery. It was so strong that it pierced though my flat affect. At first I couldn't identify what the feeling was because I had never felt it before.

It was a twinge of deep shame.

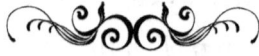

It's Not Over Yet

Dazhoni

My left fingers quivered uncontrollably as I held the pencil and practiced writing my name over and over. Sometimes it leapt out of my grasp, so I would switch to my right hand.

I wrote my name eight times; the last one was my best. I set the sheet of paper aside and grabbed my half-finished drawing, sliding the tub of crayons closer to me.

I shivered as I gently kicked my chair legs. It was another hot and humid day in July, but I felt cold. Mom said it was because of all the weight I had lost; I was twenty pounds lighter than when I had gone in for my operation. That's why Mom made sure there was a bottle of chocolate drink on the dining room table across from me.

The house was especially quiet.

Shundiin was staying at my Aunt Vicky's for the week. There was a summer theatre troupe that she, Katie and I had joined last summer, but I was obviously too sick to be part of it this year. She and Katie were probably at rehearsal right now.

I drew four purple, squiggly lines on the paper. They were the arms and legs of an orange, chicken nugget-shaped lump. Off to the side I drew a black box with two circles: a boombox; I added musical notes floating above it. *Jimmy the Dancing Tumor.*

Of course, I now realized how serious the tumor was, but I missed being and feeling like my old silly self. Slowly but surely, my emotions and sense of humor were coming back. Even though I was still nauseous all the time, I was no longer throwing up every day. And I didn't want to lie in bed all the time, either. I was learning how to get around the home on my own, by guiding my hands along the walls, furniture, anything within arm's reach.

This week, Dad and I had finished watching *The Lord of the Rings*. Dad said I was like Frodo, the Ring Bearer, because I also had a heavy burden to carry. Frodo had to take the ring on a difficult journey all the way to Mordor. Just like I had to make the journey all the way to getting better.

At least the surgery and the first few weeks of recovery were over. I was on the mend, little by little. Maybe by the time school started again in September I would be all better, and I could live my life as if none of this had happened.

"Dazhoni, can we talk to you?" It was Mom's voice.

I slowly lifted my head. I hadn't heard my parents walk in. "Okay."

The picture was mostly finished. As I stuffed the crayons back into the container, my left hand twitched as I attempted to hold the box steady.

"Do you remember when we went to the appointment in Fargo last week and the doctor talked about radiation treatments?" Mom asked.

I shrugged.

Mom once again explained that I would be getting a treatment to kill the remaining cancer cells in my brain. It would last several weeks, and I would begin sessions in another month, once I've recovered more.

"Will it hurt?"

"I don't know." She peered over at Dad who simply looked at me without an answer.

"Will it make me sick?"

Mom didn't reply, so Dad said, "Honey, we don't know. Different people have different reactions. But yes, it could make you sick for a short while. But it's very important that you have the treatment to kill any remaining cancer cells."

My throat tightened and I didn't want to hear about it anymore. What if getting radiation meant that I wasn't going to be all better by the time school started? Then I remembered the part in the Lord of the Rings movie where Frodo had brought the ring to a place called Rivendell; he had thought that the worst was over and that his journey was done. But the ring wasn't safe there. He had found out that there was still a long way to go.

My lip quivered. Radiation treatment meant that this journey wasn't over, not even close. I was only at Rivendell.

It felt good to have tears running down my cheeks. They were my first since my surgery. It felt good to remember that there was a girl inside this zombie self, even if she was sad and afraid. Looking into my parents' faces, I knew I had to be brave, like Frodo.

"I don't think I'm going to like this adventure."

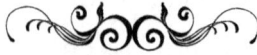

Why Me?

One long-term side effect will be memory loss.

Brushing away the tears welling up in my eyes, my feet tripped over each other. I held out my arms to help me keep balance as I started to run.

"You can't be running!"

I ignored Mom shouting after me as she stepped out of the Jeep. I didn't look back.

There will be long-term effects to the brain from the radiation. She will later experience some memory loss ...

Passing the neighbor's house, I didn't know where I was going, I just knew I had to get away. Away from what the radiologist had said at our appointment, away from what was now my life.

During this week I had realized that my flat-effect was wearing off. I was beginning to feel, and now I was feeling despair. I was devastated by everything that had happened to me and by what was yet to come.

Memory loss.

At first I had tried to joke about it as I walked out of the clinic in Fargo. Using an adult voice, I had asked Mom and Shundiin who they were, pretending I couldn't remember anything. But by the time we got to the Jeep my real feelings came bubbling out. I cried the entire way home.

My sneakers pounded away on the pavement. I decided to take the path Dad and I walked, except starting from the opposite direction. I made a right turn - or tried to. Not wearing my eye patch, I saw the trees and houses double and split downwards when my knees hit the sidewalk. Hard.

Argh!

I wanted to scream. Feeling dizzy, I slowly climbed to my feet. I hated everything the surgery had done to me. What had the doctors been thinking? Why hadn't they just left the tumor in my head and given me a life supply of Excedrin? Taking Excedrin every few hours for the rest of my life would be better than all this. Sniffling, I continued down the empty street where the elderly couple and painted gnomes lived.

How could this have happened to me? I was just a kid. Every other kid I knew had never gotten sick like this.

Then another thought hit me like a punch to the stomach. *That's because other kids don't have anger problems like me.*

Had the tumor formed because of my temper, and all the times I had yelled at my mom and my sister? Had the cells in my brain turned angry and cancerous because of me? *Is it my fault that I have cancer?*

Zig-zagging up the street, I had the urge to run again.

"Hey! Dazhoni!"

Flustered, I managed to keep my balance as I turned around in time for a bike to skid to a stop right in front of me. I knew that dirt bike anywhere. Cody.

"Dazhoni! Where have you been?" he said. I slowly lifted my head to look straight into his round face. "And where's your bike?"

Across the street behind him was the bottom of the hill where we had ridden our bikes only weeks earlier. It felt like it had been years ago. Everything had changed now. At a loss for words, I looked through his smudged glasses, into his eyes. What could I say? How do I explain everything?

"Uh . . . I've been sick," I finally replied. "I had surgery and I've lost my balance."

"Yeah, you seem different." Cody scrutinized me with his owl-like eyes.

I thought he got it. That my world had been pulled out from beneath my feet. I was a different girl than the one who had raced down the hill with him.

Without warning, he knuckled my shoulder. I staggered backwards as my arms flailed.

"Whoa. That's weird!"

Weird? He didn't get it. Changing the subject, he began telling me about something, something totally outside my world of circumstances and something I could not care less about. I just stood there, hunkered into my own thoughts, my own world. My *weird* world.

"I have to go," I said, hoping I wasn't being too abrupt. I awkwardly waved and trudged away, drained of my frustration, drained of anger. Finally making it to my front door, I was relieved to be alone.

"When will you get to ride your bike again?' I heard him call after me.

I escaped through the front door and pretended not to hear him. Back in my room, I let the tears flow.

I didn't know when I would be able to ride my bike again. I didn't know what radiation was going to do to me. And I certainly didn't know when I would get to be a normal kid again, talking about normal kid things. Cody couldn't understand that. No one could.

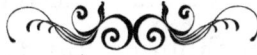

Kamp KACE

"Welcome, girls!" A heavyset woman with dark, curly hair beamed at my sister and me from the other side of the check-in table. She and two other adults wore blue T-shirts with the words **KAMP KACE** stamped across the front in bold, white letters. Although I was just meeting her, I knew her heart was as warm as her smile.

"Do you two know what Kamp KACE stands for?" she asked. She pronounced it as Kay-cee.

Both Shundiin and I shook our heads.

"It stands for Kids Against Cancer Everywhere!"

Mom kissed us goodbye and I heard her whisper to Shundiin, "Take care of your sister."

I lifted my face towards the trees. The weight of my backpack and sleeping bag began to make my knees shake, but I didn't mind. I had believed that

I was the only kid in the world that had cancer, but here was proof that I wasn't. Mom had heard about a week-long camp for kids like me - kids that have or have had cancer. Siblings could go, too. I was glad Shundiin was here with me; she would be my steady arm, and I would stick to her like glue!

"What will we do there?" I had asked Mom while packing my bag. If all the kids were as sick as I was, would everyone just be lying around most of the days? Watching movies, perhaps?

"See that cabin over there?" another lady said. She had fire red hair and was looking directly at me. "It has other girls that are around your age. And that one - " she pointed and looked at Shundiin, "has girls your age. At your cabins, change into your swimsuits and come back here so you can take the swim test. Okay?"

Shundiin and I exchanged glances. I could tell that she, too, was disappointed that we weren't going to be in the same cabin. We lugged our stuff to our separate cabins and promised to meet each other back at the top of the hill before going down to the lake.

The other girls must already be taking the swim test, I thought as I stepped into the quiet cabin. I set my bags at the foot of an empty bunk bed, then sat down to change. I covered an eye so that I could focus on the zipper on my backpack. Not wanting to look any weirder than I already did with my lopsided gait, I had decided to leave my eyepatch at home. I really didn't want to change into my swimsuit; I felt too dizzy to swim. But that was probably how all the other kids felt, too.

When I met up with my sister, she held out her arm for me the way Dad had shown her. I already missed Dad. We had had to say good-bye to him before coming here, and he was probably already on his flight back to China. He had cried and hugged me tightly just hours ago. "It's the hardest time I've ever had leaving you guys, but I have to keep my job so I'm able to support you."

Good thing I was here, so I wouldn't spend the rest of the day in my room feeling sad. The slope was steep, and Shundiin was having a difficult time helping me keep my balance; I felt like crawling down the hill instead. Finally reaching the bottom, I felt a lurching in my stomach. I hadn't expected there to be so many kids. As I followed my sister, we made our way through the crowd of smiling, laughing boys and girls. There were kids younger than Shundiin, and there were teens here, too. A group of them were playfully shoving each other into the water when the life guard wasn't looking.

They all looked so healthy. Did they really have cancer like me?

When we got to the end of the line, a tall girl in a blue bikini immediately spun around. "Hi! I'm Megan! I saw you guys getting checked in earlier and I think you're in my cabin. What's your name?"

"Dazhoni." For a long, awkward moment I realized how flat my tone still sounded, and I wondered if it made her uncomfortable. My emotionless face probably didn't help, either. I consciously forced myself to smile.

"I also noticed the scar on the back of your head. Do you have brain cancer?"

I nodded, self-consciously reaching my hand up to the back of my head. The stitches had dissolved, but there was a thick, silky scar as evidence.

"I used to have lung cancer," Megan said, pointing to the white lines on her torso. "I had to get a whole lung taken out," she continued matter-of-factly. "Then the cancer spread, so I had to get part of this one taken out, too."

I stared at her scars. I had never heard of something like that happening to a kid before! How are you even breathing? I wondered.

The line moved forward, but Megan was too busy talking to notice. "I used to have long, straight hair like you guys, but chemo made it all fall out. And you know what? It grew back curly! Isn't that cool?"

A whistle blew. The line in front of us was gone, and it was Megan's turn to swim to the buoys and back. She spun around in surprise.

Looking at the other kids, I figured that I had to be one of the sickest ones here. But I also realized something else as I watched Megan charge into the lake: I wasn't the only one anymore.

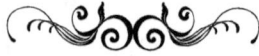

KACE Coolness

"You look like you could use a little help. Want a lift?"

All of the other campers were far ahead of me, and I had lost Shundiin. As I concentrated on keeping my balance, I was trailing behind everyone. When the golf cart pulled up, I hoped it would pass me, too, so I was embarrassed when it stopped right next to me.

"Hop in!"

Squinting at him in the bright sunlight, I recognized the piercings and tattoos. He was one of the camp leaders at the swimming test yesterday. He had the coolest Mohawk.

"Thanks," I said, as I sat down next to him. I had never ridden in a golf cart before.

"Hey, no problem! I'll give you a ride anytime I see you. Now, hold on, it gets a little bumpy!"

Hold onto what? I wondered, quickly grabbing ahold of the seat when we started to move. He was right, it was bumpy!

The light breeze caused me to shudder beneath my baggy black hoodie. It had to be almost ninety degrees, but a camp leader in the cafeteria had handed me her hoodie when she noticed me shivering. Right afterwards, an announcement came that we would all be making the trek to the other side of the campground to take part in some activities.

It was a long grassy path. We were quickly catching up to a group of kids and camp leaders up ahead! With the wind in my hair and a thrill in my chest, it kind of reminded me of being on my bike again.

"Look! It's Dazhoni!"

"Whoa! She gets to ride in the cart!"

We were passing a lot of kids; I recognized some of them were from my cabin. I had let them run past me when we had left the cafeteria so they wouldn't see me awkwardly tottering as I walked. But I didn't feel ashamed that they were seeing me now!

My face made a huge smile – all by itself. I didn't have to consciously force it.

The kids and leaders turned around to face me, stretching out their arms out so they could give me high-fives as our cart drove past them. Minutes later, we came to a stop, and as I stepped down, I noticed that we were some of the first ones there. I looked back at the camp leader, grateful beyond words for what he had done for me.

"You're a rock star!" he said as he pulled away.

⁓⟡⟡⟡⁓

Dear God. Please, please don't let me throw up. Just help me make it one more day. Please.

I had woken up dry-heaving, and I didn't know what to do if I actually threw up; the restrooms were far away from my cabin. I buried my face into my pillow, hiding it from the other girls. If I could manage to not throw up today, I would have made it through the whole week. Early morning nausea was always the worst, but it usually got better by mid-morning.

The episode finally passed, and a couple hours later I made eye contact with Shundiin in the meeting room. I pushed my way through the crowded lodge to a fold-out chair next to hers. Finally! I was with my sister again. It was the end of our time here and Mom would be picking us up soon.

A booming voice filled the room: "Let's all take a seat so we can get the award ceremony started!"

Soon a boy's name was announced: he stepped up to the camp leader and she handed him a laminated sheet of paper. He had won the most sports games. All of us clapped.

Over this week, I had missed out on many of the fun activities, like sports events and other games. I had felt too sick. But I told myself that was okay. I was probably the sickest kid here, so I wasn't going to be mad at myself for not doing enough to compete for an award.

As more names were called out, I thought about all the good things that had happened this week. I had had a great time. One of my favorite activities had been celebrating a different holiday each day of the week. The first night had been Halloween, and all the campers went trick-or-treating at the cabins. I had also enjoyed the Easter egg hunt the other day, even though I had been too nauseous to finish.

"This next award goes to these campers, who, rain or shine, never failed to get up every morning to take the polar bear plunge into the lake. Let's give them a round of applause!"

My clapping was drowned out by a thunder of cheers as the names of the polar bear plungers were read. If I had to be sick somewhere, I thought,

I'm glad it was here: a place where kids and adults understood me and made me feel comfortable with myself. I had gotten so many rides in the golf cart and so many high-fives; I had felt like a superstar every time.

The room grew quiet again in anticipation of the next boy or girl who would be called up to the front. I leaned back, ready to give my next applause.

"This next award goes to a camper, who, despite feeling poorly on many of the days, and who was at the nurse's station during many of our events, always kept a positive attitude, never complained, and always showed appreciation for even the smallest gestures of kindness. This is the *Biggest Trooper Award*, and it goes to - drum roll please . . . Dazhoni Green!"

I froze, hardly believing my ears. It had to be a mistake. Heads turned in my direction and there was some awkward shuffling about in the room. They were waiting for me to stand up, and I was waiting for the camp leader to read out the correct name. "Go up!" Shundiin finally whispered, nudging me.

Not knowing what else to do, I hesitantly stood up and made my way to the front of the room. The woman met me halfway and wrapped me in a hug before handing me the laminated sheet of paper. It wasn't a mistake. My name was written right in the center. The room filled with cheers. I glanced up to find my sister, and noticed Megan in another row, also clapping. Off to the right, the camp leader with the Mohawk smiled broadly and gave me a thumbs-up.

Finally accepting the award, I realized that it wasn't a mistake. I knew my face was glowing, even more than it did on the day that I had won the girls' pull-ups competition in P.E. class.

This is what Kamp KACE did for me. It took away my shame and made me feel like a cool kid again.

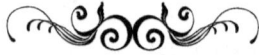

A Faithful Friend

I wiped my face as I opened my bedroom door. Even though I had rinsed my mouth, I could still taste the throw up. I was nauseous to the point of vomiting, but I still wanted to finish the game of Monopoly.

I crept into the living room. Sunlight peeked through the curtains like it couldn't wait to pour inside.

It must be around eight o'clock, I thought. I balanced myself by reaching out to each piece of furniture along my way. On the carpet lay the board game. At one end, Monopoly money and property cards were stacked in neat piles; at the other end, everything was haphazardly scattered about. That was my side.

It had been my birthday yesterday. I had felt too sick to have any cake, but Mom had insisted on inviting AJ for a sleepover anyway. I had tried to convince her not to. I hadn't wanted AJ to see me like this. I wasn't at Kamp KACE anymore, and kids in the normal world didn't understand.

But AJ ended up sleeping over and playing Monopoly with me. She liked to strategize, only buying the higher valued property squares. I just bought anything and everything I landed on. Maybe that's why she always won.

I made my way to Shundiin's room. It was strange, but I missed her already.

AJ was lying flat on her back, her head tilted to the side, her eyes closed.

Standing over her, I poked her on her shoulder. "Hey, wake up," I whispered. "Want to finish the game?" Mom was still sleeping and I didn't want to wake her.

AJ's eyes opened instantly and she jumped out of bed. She held my arm, supporting my balance, and we quietly entered the living room. This would probably be our last game for a while.

Mom had made two major decisions. First, I would be going back to Mayo to get radiation. Mom thought it would be best to have doctors who already knew me. We would be leaving in a week or so.

Her second major decision was about Shundiin: she would live in Iowa for the time Mom and I would be in Rochester. My older cousin, Jennifer, and her husband,

Kendall, had offered to take her into their home so that Mom could focus on taking care of me. She would start school there, and live with second cousins, Zachary and Jeremy. Shundiin had really cried when she left; she had never been away from Mom for such a long time.

AJ and I sprawled out on the floor and continued our game. My left arm was still shaky. I accidentally dropped the dice a couple times because my fingers still twitched when I attempted careful movements. I was embarrassed at first, but AJ acted like she didn't even notice. She talked to me and treated me the same way she had before my surgery. Joking and making me laugh, it was just like old times; it was comfortable being with her. I felt a twinge of guilt for not wanting her to come over and see me.

"Welcome! Welcome!" AJ greeted as I landed on her property. I handed over some Monopoly bills. "Thank you! Come again!" It cracked me up every time.

Even though I was different now, AJ didn't treat me any differently. Our game ended with all my properties being mortgaged. I realized that she didn't need to fully understand what I was going through; she was my dear friend who always cared about me, and not even cancer could change that.

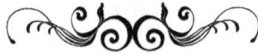

The Comfort Inn

September

A man with a giant slug creature inside his back is butchered with an axe by one of the evil townspeople. Menacingly, they surround their next victim. She can't escape. She will be next.

I desperately reached for the remote and pressed the red power button to *Off*.

Goosebumps ran down my arms, like tiny slug eggs were inside them. I shuddered, shaking the thought from my head. Why did I watch that scary movie? Wasn't my concern about starting radiation enough to be worried about?

I walked over to the large window and pushed away the shades, allowing light to shine through. I was hoping to see our Jeep pull into the parking lot down below. The hotel room suddenly felt creepy, and I didn't want to be alone in here any longer.

Scary movies gave me nightmares, and I wasn't supposed to watch them. Most kids I knew didn't rat on themselves, but I always did, and I knew Mom was going to be mad when I told her.

Mom had left to get some groceries; we were going to stay here until a room opened at the Ronald McDonald House. Trying to distract my mind from slugs with sharp teeth and axe murderers, I lifted my math textbook out of my backpack and threw my notebook and pencil onto the bed. Right before we had left Rothsay, I had gone with Mom to school to meet with my sixth-grade teacher, Mrs. Tillman. She was nice. I was given textbooks and worksheets that Mom could help me with while we were in Rochester. By working on the assignments a couple of hours a day, I figured I could keep up with a lot of what the class was doing.

Lying on my stomach, I wrote out the problems for Chapter Three. I noticed a difference in how I felt each new month. Even my handwriting was looking smoother. Yet all of a sudden, the image of that slug returned; it had crippled the man and made him so sick. Kind of like what cancer was doing to me.

An image of a cancerous tumor with gnashing teeth popped into my head as I looked up from my textbook. I kept thinking about it; comparing myself to that man with the slug inside him. I felt like I was in a horror movie.

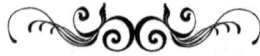

Home Away From Home

The alien dipped the needle into ink before jabbing it into my head in three different places. With her scaly, green fingers, she held up a perforated mask; it kind of looked like a scary hockey mask.

"This is it," she said. I held my breath as she held it up to my face.

Actually, she wasn't a scary alien, but a very nice technician who was fitting me for my radiation mask. I had felt so cool when she had told me that those were *real* tattoos that she had inked onto my head. I couldn't contain myself when I had shown them to Mom in the waiting room. I pushed away the hair above my ears and above the scar at the back of my skull. "I have real tattoos!" I ignored her when she replied that the dots were almost too small to see. At the parking ramp, I had lowered my voice and excitedly asked, "Are my tattoos *illegal*? I'm just a kid."

She only sighed.

We soon arrived at the Ronald McDonald House where a room had opened up for us. The first thing I noticed as I stepped out of the Jeep was a big red heart painted on the top window of the building, something I hadn't noticed when we had been here the night before my surgery.

When we entered, a woman at the desk told us that she would be giving us a tour. It was going to be our home for a while. Suddenly feeling shy, I stepped behind Mom as she introduced us, then we followed her through the lobby. As I looked around, I vaguely remembered the model train set in the center; miniature railroad tracks circled about. Our guide showed us the community room, the computer room, and the mail cubbies. I grabbed Mom's hand and squeezed it when we stopped in front of the Game Room. Peering through the window, I could see video games and arcade-like machines. I couldn't wait to go in there!

"The second and third floors are the rooms for the families," she explained as we neared the elevator. "Rooms on both floors share kitchens, snack bars, lounge areas, and a couple play rooms." Mom was handed a key and I was anxious to see our room.

"We're in room 307," Mom said.

"Which floor?"

Mom chuckled as we stepped out of the elevator. "Third floor, Silly."

"Your room is that way." The lady gestured to the left. "But first, I want to show you something special."

We followed her down the brightly carpeted hallway, and Mom smiled knowingly. *What does she know that I don't know?*

"Here's the kitchen, and the surprise," the woman said, pointing at the window.

I gazed past the tables and refrigerators and there it was! "Mom, it's the heart! The one we saw from the parking lot!" The huge red heart looked even bigger from here. As I stood there admiring it, my shyness faded away and I couldn't help but smile.

"I knew you'd like it," the lady said, smiling back at me.

I was so happy that Mom and I were going to stay here while I received my radiation treatments. Even though we had only been here for a short while, the Ronald McDonald House already felt like home.

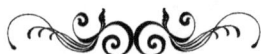

A Lucky Girl

I had never seen a yellow baby before.

I hadn't known that there was such a thing as a sickness that could make your skin and eyes turn yellow. And I had never heard the word *jaundice* before. Mom had explained it to me after we had seen a dark-haired woman pushing a blue stroller on our floor.

"You're Navajo?" Mom asked after our introductions were made. I braced myself for the story I've heard a million times.

"We were teachers on a Navajo Indian Reservation in Arizona for ten years, so we gave our girls Navajo names." She never explained that *we* meant Dad and her. "This is Dazhoni. And my other daughter is Shundiin. This one, by the time she was four years old, believed she was Navajo. She once said to me, 'I'm brown, you're white; I'm Navajo, you're not!' Eventually, we moved back to Minnesota, a bit concerned that she was losing her identity."

They both laughed. We hadn't even been here a week and Mom had already made friends with almost everyone on our floor.

"Her pre-school teachers said that she spoke better Navajo than the Navajo children! Dazhoni, why don't you count one through ten in Navajo for her?"

This is when I'd get shy. I tightly pressed my lips shut to make sure no words would come out.

"Go on."

Nope.

"Please!"

I shook my head, beginning to feel embarrassed.

Giving up, Mom rolled her eyes at me. "Well anyway, it's so nice meeting you and your little one!"

The Navajo mom pushed her stroller past us, and I glanced one more time at the baby with the pudgy, yellow face, tucked comfortably within a flowery blanket.

It was back to homework for me. Mom read off another reading comprehension question from a boring sailboat story, and I playfully groaned. We were sitting at a small table outside our room, and worksheets were scattered across the table. I pretended to hate working on school stuff with Mom, but I actually looked forward to it. It made me feel like a regular kid, and acting like I thought homework was boring made me feel even more normal.

My first week of radiation had been a breeze. The appointments were at two o'clock every day, Monday through Friday. They were scheduled so I would have my weekends free; that way, I could recoup before the next rounds, although I hadn't had any negative effects so far. During the treatments, I would lie down on a moving table with my face buried in my mask. As the table moved, I would hear the buzzing of a machine somewhere in the room, and then, *Presto!* It was over! It hadn't hurt, and it hadn't made me feel sicker. I had been nervous and worried for nothing.

I sat up straight and tried to focus on the question Mom read aloud. Suddenly, there was the shuffling of approaching footsteps, and we shifted our attention back down the hallway; two huddled figures were coming our way. A man and a girl almost as tall as him. I looked over at Mom.

"Dazhoni, do you remember when I mentioned to you that there was another child staying here who has an ependymoma tumor like you had?"

I thought for a moment, then nodded.

"Well, that's her and her father," Mom whispered. "They're from Minnesota, the Detroit Lakes area."

The man was tall and stocky. His arm was wrapped around the girl, supporting her as they walked. She was skinny, blond, and pretty. As they drew closer, I noticed that she was slouching, and one of her eyes was closed.

"She has the same type of cancer as you," Mom continued to whisper. "Except her tumor is in an inoperable area of her brain stem."

"What's that mean?"

"Shhh!"

"Sorry," I said in a quieter voice. I'd never been very good at whispering. "What's *inoperable* mean?"

"It means she can't have surgery."

As they solemnly lumbered towards our table, I lifted my hand and gave them a small wave. Why do they look sad? They should be happy that she won't have to have surgery. The effects of surgery felt far worse than having the tumor, I thought. She was lucky.

The father forced a grim smile, but neither of them waved back as they continued past us.

I saw her dad one more time after that, then I never saw either of them again. At the time, I never really gave it another thought; I had figured that she had gotten well and returned home. Several years later, Mom told me the rest of the story. The girl hadn't been lucky at all. She had died.

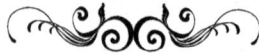

Goosebumps

I shielded my eyes before allowing them to adjust to the light. As stealthily as I could manage, I let our door click shut.

It was two in the morning, and I still couldn't fall asleep. This had happened last night, too. But I made up my mind that I wouldn't toss and turn all night again, so I quietly escaped. I didn't remember my glasses until after I shut the door behind me.

I was wearing my new pajama pants that Aunt Sandy had sent me. They were red, with little yellow dogs on them, but without my glasses on they looked like little yellow, blurry splotches.

Not sure of what I was going to do, I crept past a couple of tables, over to the bookcases in the lounge area. On one side of the giant TV were movies. I noticed *Monster's Inc* right away, but because it was night time, I figured it would be rude to have any noise on. At the other side of the TV was a bookshelf. I squinted to read the titles.

My latest MRI showed that I had fluid built up in my brain, so I had to take steroids: monster pills that made me choke every time I had to swallow one. Since the day I had started taking them I've had trouble falling asleep. As I skimmed through the book titles, I again landed on the entire series that took up a portion of the middle shelf. *Goosebumps*.

I picked one out and examined the cover. *Night of the Living Dummy*. Ever since fourth grade I had wanted to read *Goosebumps*. Other kids in my class borrowed them from the school library, but not me. Mom had said no; they were too scary, so I wasn't allowed to read them.

I clutched the softcover book in my hands and found a comfortable spot on the couch. This was one of my favorite places outside our room. I held the book up close to my face with one hand, and covered an eye with the other. I didn't notice the double vision as much anymore, only when I tilted my head or became tired. And even though I couldn't fall asleep, I felt exhausted. This was just a small setback; I had told myself. Once I was off the monster pills,

I'd be feeling better again. I was also in the middle of Week Two of radiation, and it was still easy. If it was doing anything at all, I couldn't feel it.

So tonight I had waited to hear Mom snoring before sneaking out to read another *Goosebumps* book. Mom had been wrong. They weren't too scary.

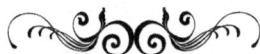

Zach

"Do you want to go downstairs to the Game Room?"

I turned to Mom and she gave me the okay. "Sure," I told Zach as we headed towards the door.

I had met Zach and his mom in the shared kitchen a few days ago. Several families on our floor had met for lunch, and I had ended up sitting next to a boy who had come all the way from Greece to have surgery on his leg. The Navajo mother and her baby were there, too. Another girl I had met was also there. Her name was Jayne; she was seventeen, and she had something wrong with her digestive tract. I had poured her a glass of Gatorade, but she had told me she couldn't drink it like that; she had poured half of it back, then diluted hers with water.

By the time Zach and his mom had arrived, the food was gone and almost everyone had left. They had just completed their tour of the house. What I had first noticed about Zach was that he had brown hair and glasses, just like me. We were also the same height. His mom had even commented: "You two could pass as brother and sister!"

I learned that he had a heart disease. As we had talked, I noticed thin, black shoulder straps supporting a backpack that he wore. It was something that I really hadn't thought about much until seeing him again today.

Why is he still wearing that backpack?

I followed Zach down the hallway and to the stairs, and I was able to examine him without his noticing. The backpack was small and very plain looking; it didn't have a lot of zippers or colorful pockets like the one I had. It was dark green and I only counted one zipper.

I paused at the stairs as Zach stomped his way down. Stairs were the most difficult for me; my vertigo and double vision went into overdrive. Maybe I should've used the elevator. I cautiously took one step at a time, grasping the rail tightly. *You have nothing to be ashamed of.* I reminded myself of what Dad had said, but I couldn't help it. I didn't want Zach to see me like this.

Once I reached the mailboxes, I caught a glimpse of the green backpack before my new friend vanished around a corner. I noticed something about the backpack that I hadn't before; a tube stuck out from an opening on the pack, and it dropped down and looped up inside the front of his shirt. The tube attaches to his body, I discovered, feeling like a detective. That meant the backpack was something medical related. But what was inside the backpack? And what was that tube for?

Opening the door to the Game Room, I saw that Zach was already seated at one end of the couch, just as the *Kim Possible* theme song began playing on the Disney Channel. Walking past the foosball table, I noticed a PlayStation 2 under the TV stand. On the floor was a *LEGO Star Wars* game that hadn't been put away.

I sat down next to Zach. A couple minutes into the show, I caught something out of the corner of my eye: Zach had turned away and had lifted up his shirt, then quickly pulled it back down. *He's checking the tube.* I just knew it! But where was it attached on his body?

A few minutes later, he checked it again, and I was able to continue my investigation. As he lifted up his shirt, I leaned forward to see better, hoping to find some answers. But in that instant, I learned everything I needed to know. I didn't see anything; as soon as I had turned my head, Zach noticed me watching and immediately put his shirt down. I quickly turned away, but not before I saw his hurt expression directed towards me.

For the rest of the show, Zach didn't check on the tube. And for the rest of the show, I sat there feeling bad. I never found out where the tube was attached, or why Zach needed the backpack. Yet at that one moment, I had lost the urge of needing to know. I had found out how it made him feel, and why he didn't want me to see.

It made him feel ashamed.

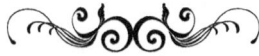

Staying Positive

I don't know how you do it. A family friend had written to me in the email Mom read.

With labored steps, I kicked a damp pile of blurry red, yellow and orange out of my way. Leaves blanketed most of the sidewalk. The air was heavy and earthy. Mom had a firm grip on my arm, and we had almost completed a circle around the Ronald McDonald House late this morning. Light was seeping through the branches above our heads. The sun was out, but I couldn't feel its warmth.

I had vomited after waking up this morning. My nausea was getting worse, and I was having difficulty eating. I didn't want to believe it was from my radiation treatments, but one of my therapists had said these were normal side effects from having radiation to the brain. I also had a dry mouth and a sour, metallic taste that wouldn't go away. My spit was as thick as rope, so Mom had bought me hard candies to suck on throughout the day. That helped a bit. I popped one into my mouth as we continued on our walk.

We had been talking about our time seeing my cousin Jennifer earlier this week. She had come up from Iowa to visit us. Shundiin was adjusting well to her new living arrangements; she had even joined the soccer team at her school. Jennifer told us a funny story about my little second cousin, Zachary, who had told someone that I was in Rochester *getting gunk out of my head.*

Mom began talking about all the support we were getting from family and friends, including all the encouraging emails and *Get Well* cards that we loved reading together. The Ronald McDonald House was only a few minutes away when I abruptly stopped and listened. Whistling. I recognized the silly tune. Gazing upwards, I excitedly nudged Mom and pointed to a figure on a rooftop. "Look!"

I had learned that song when I was at Kamp KACE. I mouthed the words in harmony with the man's whistling. "I don't wanna be a chicken, I don't wanna be a duck, so I shake my butt!" I made my hands into beaks, opening and closing them. Mom shook her head, but she couldn't hide a tiny smile. I giggled the rest of the way back to our building.

As soon as we entered, we stopped by our mail cubby. Peering inside, I spotted whiskers and triangle-shaped ears. I pulled out a fluffy, gray tabby cat wearing a red, heart-shaped tag.

"Aww, so cute!" I hugged it tightly.

Every Friday, someone at the Ronald McDonald House placed a Beanie Baby in the cubbies for each family. By now, I had a handful of them. They sat on the top bunk with me, keeping me company on mornings I felt too sick to get out of bed.

I was learning to have a new outlook on my daily life; I kept an eye out for all the positive moments, whatever made me laugh or smile. The *good* things. That's what I would now focus on. All the little good things that made the big hard things easier. Like a new Beanie Baby. I felt like my heart was lighting up the entire first floor of the Ronald McDonald House.

This is how you do it, I thought in response to the email Mom had read.

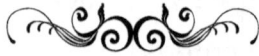

Another Reality Check

"Don't overfill the tub this time!" Mom shouted out from the other side of the door. At least that's what it sounded like amid the crashing, rushing water.

I flinched as I turned off the faucet, then slowly stepped into the frothy bubbles. My left arm was still sore. Holding onto the handicap bar for balance, I slid myself deeper into my bath. A knee almost knocked over the little green jug of bubble bath lying on the edge of the tub. It had an image of a smiling watermelon in the center, and I had just used up the last of the soap.

Suds now reached the faucet, making the tub seem fuller than it really was. I rested my bruised arm on the porcelain ledge, being careful to not get it wet, especially where a section of the IV tube was taped down and wrapped in cellophane. I didn't mind that the needle had been left in my arm, because that meant I wouldn't have to get poked again tomorrow.

I looked forward to these bubble baths. I took one every evening after returning from a busy day of doctor appointments and radiation treatments. I happily hummed to a song stuck in my head. I had watched several episodes of *Phil of the Future* on the Disney Channel while getting my IV fluids, and the silly song from the show played over and over in my brain.

"You have tiny veins like many cancer patients," the nurse had said. I could tell she felt bad when the third vein she tried also popped. She apologized over and over.

"It's okay." I hadn't wanted her to feel bad. I was getting pretty used to it by now; the needles didn't bother me. The discomfort they caused hardly compared to the other things I was going through. On her fourth try she had finally managed to fit the needle in properly, and she told me she would leave it for when I came back tomorrow.

I smeared suds onto my face, giving myself a bubble beard, and waited for the water to look less soapy before dunking my head. Blocking my nose, I submerged my entire body, feeling my hair fan out beneath the water's surface.

I was afraid to touch my hair. Lately, I had been waking up to find small patches of it on my pillow. I touched my temples and the area above my scar at the base of my skull; it hurt like a sun-burn, but I couldn't feel any more smooth spots. One of my radiation therapists had explained that I would feel sun-burnt on the areas being treated. I would also experience hair loss. That part scared me; I didn't want to lose my hair. Luckily, the strands that were falling out must be too few to be noticeable. Still, I tried not to touch my hair too much.

"Phil, Ph-i-il of the Future . . . " I sang after sitting up again. I rubbed the water away from my eyes and gazed down at the dark blots swimming in my bathwater.

I blinked. The water really was darker. Had my hair been that dirty? Pushing soapy bubbles away from my eyes, I peered deeper into the water. I scooped up some of the dark, spidery pieces; long strands of hair slipped through my fingers. It wasn't dirt. It was my hair!

There had to be hundreds of strands floating in the tub, like dark webs of seaweed. There was no way it could no longer be unnoticeable on my head. I frantically rubbed at my temples and the spot above my scar; there were no bald patches that I could feel. I moved my hands around my entire scalp, and I found it. On the crown of my head I could feel a smooth patch of skin the size of a half dollar. The hair around it felt thin, so I stopped touching it so it wouldn't fall out, too.

The shock of it slowly faded like the remaining bubbles in the tub. Now I only felt like crying.

I scooped up all the hairs I could and carefully set the soggy pile on the rim of the tub. I then sat there with my arms wrapped about myself until the water grew cold. I felt so ugly.

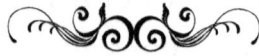

Scary Thoughts

How much longer until I'm all better?

I pushed open the heavy doors to the Ronald McDonald House with the same force I used to push away the thought. Crossing the parking lot, I began lumbering up the grassy hill that led to a small park nearby. Mom had told me not to wander off by myself, but right now I didn't care. I wanted to be alone with the troubling thoughts circling around in my head.

A sharp wind whipped against my cheeks, and the ground beneath my feet felt as hard as stone. Soon everything would be covered in snow. I finally came to an old rickety swing that I had once noticed during one of my walks with Mom. Wrapping my fingers around the cold metal chains, I sat down and pushed out with my legs, launching myself into flight.

Tonight had been the worst Halloween I ever had. I threw up all morning, and now Mom wasn't feeling well. There would be some Halloween activities going on in the community room, but I didn't want to go without her.

Kicking out at the sky, I propelled myself higher and higher. I thought back on last Halloween, when we had just moved to Hawley. Mom and Aunt Vicky had taken Katie, Shundiin, and me trick-or-treating, and I had somehow ended up with the most candy.

Now, every special day was just another day of disappointment. I was sick on the Fourth of July, on my birthday, and now on Halloween. Will I still be sick by Thanksgiving?

My lip quivered. Gripping the chains tighter, I pumped my legs harder. I was high in the air now. *What if I'm still sick when it's Christmas?* Tears splayed across my cheeks. Gazing up into the deep purple sky, an even darker thought crept into my mind. *What if I don't get better at all? What if I die?*

No! With that, I leapt off the swing and hit the ground with a thud. *That could never happen! I'm just a kid!* I swiped away my tears and brushed off my sweatpants. I simply had to be better by

Christmas. I just *had* to. My fingers were numb with cold, so I started back towards the Ronald McDonald House.

I was hoping to slink back inside unnoticed, but that didn't happen. Through the doors, I saw the Navajo mother leaning over her baby's stroller by the mail cubbies. Our eyes met and I hoped she couldn't tell that I had been crying.

"How are you feeling?" she asked me as I entered.

"Fine," I said with an attempted smile. I drew closer so I could peer into the stroller.

"I'm so relieved! My baby received her liver transplant," she said, hardly above a whisper. "Now she's just sleeping a lot."

I peered down into the stroller, barely able to make out the tiny, yellowish face half-hidden among the layers of fleece blankets. She looked so peaceful. I knew that sleeping was a good thing; it meant the body was healing.

"Oh, wow!" I replied, trying to act surprised. But Mom had already told me. They couldn't keep waiting for a baby-sized liver, so she was given a section of an adult liver instead.

I chatted with the mother for a couple minutes, then pressed the *Up* arrow on the elevator panel. On my ride to the third floor, I couldn't help but wonder: *Why is the baby still that sickly yellow color? Didn't a new liver mean the yellow color would go away? Why isn't she all better by now?*

The elevator came to a stop, and the door slid open. I wobbled down the carpeted hall with my right hand held against the wall for balance. When I stepped into our room, I noticed that the lights were on and Mom was up. She looked like she was feeling a little better.

"Where were you?"

I didn't want to be in trouble, so I just shrugged and thought about the swing and then seeing the baby downstairs. I unzipped my jacket and closed the door behind me.

I was still sick, just like the Navajo baby. I guess I had to be patient. In time, both that little, yellow baby and I would get better. *After all, we're kids; and kids don't die.*

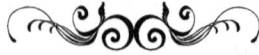

The Green Dragon

"Tie your shoe!" Mom demanded as we pushed past a carousel of coats when we stepped off the escalator. I knew Mom wouldn't stop nagging me until I did, but I couldn't squat down right in the center of the aisle of the busy mall. I wished I had noticed my shoelace when we were still in the Jeep, on our way here from the hospital.

Barnes and Noble was at the other end of the building, so we still had a ways to walk. Mom said it was my special day and she would buy me any book I wanted. Except *Goosebumps*. I had already asked her about that.

Yesterday had been my last day of radiation, and I had been transported to the center on a gurney. I had been in the hospital for a couple of days, and they had still made me go to my two o'clock radiation appointments. Mom had ridden over with me in the ambulance, which had been kind of cool.

I squeezed Mom's arm in excitement, ignoring my nausea and dizziness. What book would I get? My Uncle Lonnie had sent me *The Magician's Nephew* and *The Lion, The Witch, and the Wardrobe*. Would I get the third book in the *Chronicles of Narnia* series?

I barely noticed all the small kiosks we passed, and then something caught my eye at a shop called Games by James. I split off from Mom to get a better look. It was a large, stuffed creature that was green with gold on its belly and wings. It had white claws and purple scales of felt running down its back. A dragon. With its vibrant colors, it was the coolest one I had ever seen!

Shoppers awkwardly stepped around me as I brushed my hand down its broad head to the base of its tail. It had to be almost three feet long. Hanging around its neck was a white price tag. I had thirteen dollars in my coat pocket, but I was pretty sure that the dragon would cost way more than that. My hopes deflated as I turned the tag over. Forty-six dollars.

I didn't notice Mom until I felt her hand on my shoulder. "You really like that dragon, don't you?"

I nodded. "But it's so expensive." I felt guilty for even wanting it.

"I'll tell you what -" Mom didn't finish the rest of her sentence. I stood up, frozen, as I watched her take the stuffed creature to the store clerk and hand him her debit card.

"Thank you! Thank you!" I wrapped her in a bear hug. It was the best present ever!

"Now here's what you can do for me . . ." Mom replied sternly.

Anything! I wanted to tell her. I'd clean our room at the Ronald McDonald House if she wanted. And I would give her all my money. I grabbed my crumpled bills out of my pocket and started to hand them to her.

"Tie your shoe!"

I laughed, then bent down to comply.

On our way back to the Ronald McDonald House I decided that he was a boy dragon, and even though I couldn't think of a name for him yet, I knew exactly where I would put him.

We would be staying at the Ronald McDonald House for another month as I finished my physical therapy and other appointments. We had switched to a new room – a *long term* room a few doors down from our old one. It was larger, and it included a second room with a coffee table and a sofa. It hadn't taken long for Mom and I to move our stuff into our new place. I still had a bunkbed to myself, and I still slept on the top where I kept my puking bowl on one side of the pillow. On the other side were my Beanie Babies.

I set my dragon at the foot of my bed. I felt so happy and so proud. He stood up there strong and brave - like me. I had conquered the radiation.

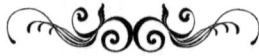

Sickness

Blood and bile.

It splashed against the inside of the toilet bowl, again, washing away the words I had scrawled onto the ceramic rim. I couldn't stop vomiting. I couldn't call out for help. I knew I was losing consciousness . . .

With my last ebb of strength, I lifted my quivering hand and pressed the pen against the filthy surface. **HELP HELP HELP** *I wrote it over and over but my disgorge always washed it away. There was no more time. I was dying. What I had to do now was tell my family that I love them.*

I LOVE -

Suddenly I heaved, and again the blood and spew washed away my letters. I lost my remaining strength and slumped to the floor. My world went black . . .

It was my recurring nightmare, but this morning it was coming true. Red vomit.

Through the blur of my tears I could make out the blood colored vomit splashed against the toilet bowl. Steadying my racing thoughts, I forced myself to think clearly. *Not blood.* Mom and I had gone out to eat with Zach and his mom last evening. I had ordered pasta with a red marinara sauce. It was only pasta sauce, I reassured myself. But that wasn't the only reason I had been reminded of my dream. Unlike all the other mornings when I had gotten sick, this time the vomiting wouldn't stop. *Am I going to die while throwing up – just like in my dream?*

Although my stomach was now empty, I kept retching. The acid climbed to the top of my throat before sliding a burning path downwards. But one thing about this morning was different than in my dream: Mom was right here with me, holding back my hair and gently rubbing my back. I wasn't alone.

When I finally stopped throwing up, Mom led me to the couch so I could lie down as she cleaned the bathroom. It was the worst sore throat that I had ever had – this dry-heaving had to stop soon. Every now and then I sat up to look at the time: six o'clock became seven o'clock, which became eight o'clock before I knew it.

Mom brought me a glass of water, but I almost immediately threw it up. She called my oncologist, the doctor that I didn't like, the one who recently took me off Zofran, my nausea medication. I had told her that although my radiation treatments were over, I still felt nauseous every day.

"Since the radiation is over, you shouldn't feel nauseous," she insisted.

"But I am!" I countered. She shook her head, obviously not believing me, and I stormed out of her office.

At least Mom believed me, and I figured the doctor finally would too, once Mom told her about this morning.

I held my breath, listening for the oncologist's response over the phone. Mom had put it on speaker:

"Well, your daughter could have the flu."

What? How can she say that? Mom and I exchanged the same look and then she hung up the phone. Gathering my coat and boots, Mom rushed me to the Out-Patient ward at St. Mary's, the place where I received my IVs every day for the radiation treatments.

Minutes later, we entered the hospital, and as Mom talked to a nurse, I vomited into a blue hospital bowl. I was soon hooked up to an IV and Mom and I were told it contained an anti-nausea medication. Within minutes the dry heaving finally stopped. At last, the acidic bile would leave my raw throat alone. I took a deep breath, grateful and relieved. The hellishness of the day was over, or so I thought.

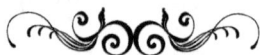

Anguish

"Sorry, Zach. She's too sick today," Mom replied after answering the door.

Sitting upright on the couch, I could see Zach's forehead and brown hair over Mom's shoulder. He had asked if I could go down to the Game Room with him. I must have looked as bad as I felt, because when Mom stepped aside, he immediately walked over and wrapped his long, baggy sleeves around me. I didn't say anything because I had lost my voice from throwing up so much.

"Feel better," he said before leaving. Mom closed the door and went back to the bedroom. I knew she was exhausted.

I was tired, too, but I didn't feel like sleeping. I didn't feel like reading or watching TV, either. I sat wrapped in my fleece blanket with Gatorade at hand on the coffee table. I also went back to what I was doing earlier: staring into nowhere and letting my thoughts wander.

What a day. And it wasn't even noon.

The room was quiet. So quiet, I could hear someone on drums at the far side of the building. *DUM. DUM. DUM. DUM.* As I listened, I could hear another sound: a woman's voice.

But wait. Those weren't drums, but shoes pounding across the floor, and the voice wasn't singing. It was wailing. A sound of piercing pain.

I heard running outside our door. Something was wrong. The cries and footsteps grew louder. I expected the running to pass, with the cries growing distant, like an ambulance passing by. But when the footsteps and cries reached their loudest, there was suddenly a loud *BANG!* My body jolted, stunned, as our entry door swung wide open.

I was looking directly into the red, puffy eyes of a woman. Black streaks of mascara ran down her cheeks and it took me a moment to recognize her. It was the Navajo mother, she had just barged right in.

Mom rushed out of the bedroom looking forlorn. For a long second that felt like forever, we just looked at each other. Then tears gushed out of the woman and she screamed: "My baby! She's dead!"

Mom let out a sharp gasp and ran to hug her as she fell to her knees.

I sat there, frozen. I couldn't fathom it. Mom was now crying, too. *It's not true,* I thought to myself as the mother's words repeated over and over in my mind.

My baby . . .

She's dead.

My baby . . . She's dead.

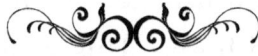

A Difficult Goodbye

"I want to give you something."

I nodded solemnly and closed the door behind me. I tried not to think about the fact that this would be the last time I'd follow Zach down the carpeted hall of the Ronald McDonald House. Instead of going down the stairs, we walked a little further and veered off into the playroom. I flipped on the light switch.

I think I had been in here once, maybe. It was a room for the little kids. Tubs of toys lined the walls; in one corner there was a tiny play stove with plastic plates and plastic, waxy looking food. At another side of the room were big, foamed cushions of different colors.

Zach tipped one over and sat down, holding his coat in his arms. As I pulled over a yellow cushion next to his red one, I could hear his mom's voice calling his name faintly in the background.

Today Zach had finished his medical treatments and he was going home. This week had been a sad one. Mom had visited with the Navajo mother all day yesterday and had given her some money. I still couldn't believe the baby was gone. Now, with Zach leaving, a selfish part of me wished he wasn't well enough yet. Mom had said that we wouldn't be going home until a few weeks from now, once all my tests were done, and when I finished my sessions of physical therapy.

My friend and I sat there, quiet for a moment. "Look, I want you to have this," he finally said. Pushing up his long sleeve, I noticed a purple band around his wrist. He took it off and dropped it in my hand. It was rubber or some kind of stretchy plastic. I ran my thumb over the letters etched across the middle. *DREAM.*

"Zach?" His mom suddenly appeared in the doorway. "There you are! I was looking all over for you. Let's go!"

"Bye," Zach quickly murmured before standing up. He threw on his coat, then gave me a half hug.

"Bye," I echoed. I watched him leave the room, giving one last look at the bulky lump beneath his coat.

I was really going to miss him. The kid with brown hair and glasses who could have passed for my brother. My Game Room buddy who had heart disease and carried a little green backpack.

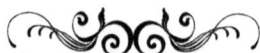

An MRI

December, 2005

Plink! Plink! Plink! Plink! Bmb. Bmb. Bmb.

Lying on my back, I was looking up through the white bars of the head coil. Pads held my head in place; and pads covered my ears. But the noise was still blaringly loud. I was used to it, though. This had to be my fourth MRI, I thought, carefully counting on my fingers without moving them.

Bmb. Bmb. Bmb.

I liked to imagine that I was in a spaceship. A spacecraft where I fit into the donut hole-shaped command center, and all the weird sounds were meteors and asteroids being blown up.

Growwwl.

That wasn't the MRI machine; it was my stomach. I wished I had eaten something before we left the Ronald McDonald House, especially since this scan wouldn't just be the usual half-hour long, but rather, an entire hour since I was having my spine scanned, too.

I tried my best not to think about my stomach and began counting Mississippi very slowly. That's how I would pass the time.

One Miss-iss-ipp-i. Two Miss-iss-ipp-i. Three Miss-iss-ipp-i.

Different rounds of noise came and went. A voice came through the ear muffs letting me know how long each sound would last. One sound lasted ten minutes, another one lasted eight. The loudest and craziest one sounded like a jackhammer breaking apart concrete.

One-hun-dred-Miss-iss-ipp-i.

Towards the end, the machine stopped, my table slid out, and a technician gave me an injection in my arm. The contrast was so they could see parts of the scan better. I could always taste it on the roof of my mouth; I thought it tasted like coldness - if coldness had a taste.

All I could think about was eating. But as the table slid back inside the tube for a final round of noises, something happened that was out of routine: the blanket that covered me became caught on some-thing, exposing my bare arms and the flimsy gown that covered my body. I knew this was bad. It was cold in here. Very cold. I held an emergency pump in one hand, but I had never squeezed it before. Was this an emergency? What if it wasn't? I just had to stiff it out until it was over. The sounds started up again.

So hungry. And *brrr!* I shuddered.

Oops. I moved.

Instead of counting, I thought about a story Mom had told me about one of the newest families that had come to stay at the Ronald McDonald House. It had been a snowy afternoon when Mom spotted a boy with a Mohawk being helped out of a car in the parking lot. As she walked closer to the House, she could see that he was holding a giant stuffed character.

"Is that Charlie Brown you're holding?" Mom asked, striking up a conversation with him.

"Yeah," he replied weakly. He had fresh stitches that ran down the side of his head and above his ear. "And after my next chemo, I'm going to get Snoopy, and then Linus, too!"

"Wow, very cool!" Mom replied.

Behind him stood a thickset figure with long, silvery curls who was still reaching into their vehicle. Always the extrovert, Mom gestured toward the adult. "Is this your grandma?" she asked.

"No," the figure replied as he turned around and faced her. He wasn't smiling through his thick beard. "I'm the *father*."

Thinking about it again, I couldn't help but giggle as I imagined how embarrassed Mom must have felt. Oops. I moved again.

The rest of the story wasn't funny, though. Mom said that the boy dropped his Charlie Brown and began vomiting in the parking lot. His father had to pick him up and carry him into the Ronald McDonald House. Mom retrieved the stuffed toy and followed them.

Brrr! Only a few minutes left, I assured myself, shivering as softly as I could. I impatiently wiggled my toes.

Then it all stopped, and the table began to move. *Yes! I'm done!* I wanted to cheer.

As I prepared to get out of the frigid machine, a technician suddenly loomed over me. He didn't remove the head coil and pads, and he didn't congratulate me.

"You've been moving too much over the last few minutes. I'm sorry, but we're going to have to start over. Now, please, stay still."

I stared at his mouth, waiting for a smile to show that he was kidding. But he adjusted the blanket, re-tucked it over my shoulders, and then the table slid back into the tube.

I wanted to cry.

It turned into another hour, the longest hour in my life. But I managed to keep still, even when I thought my stomach would start eating itself.

When I was finally done, Mom was there to save the day. I could have kissed her when she said, "I figured you'd be hungry, so I got us each a donut."

She barely finished her sentence when I snatched up a donut and devoured it.

"Whoa, you really were hungry! Do you want mine, too?"

Seizing the other glazed pastry from her hand, I gobbled that one down, too. The rumbling in my stomach stopped, and suddenly everything was okay in the world.

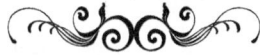

Final Tests

"Hold the door open for them!" a woman with a bob-cut instructed. A boy stood with his back firmly against the elevator door so that it wouldn't close on us. Mom pushed my wheelchair inside, then bent down to his level to thank him.

"*Ninth floor,*" declared the automated female voice. "*Going down!*"

I giggled. It never got old. Her voice dropped really low when she said that. When we took the elevator up, she would say: "*Going up!*" and her voice would raise an octave. It always made me smile, and I always looked forward to it. Especially on rough days like today.

There was a *Ding!* and Mom let the woman and boy step out first. One of my wheels jammed in the doorway gap, and she gave me an extra shove, only to have the wheelchair bump into the wall. I almost dropped the cardboard bowl I was holding. We both had to laugh as she adjusted her grip. It wasn't the first time this had happened, and it probably wouldn't be the last.

I kept my head down, near the bowl, as Mom pushed me through a sea of people on First Floor. Soon we were in another waiting room, my last appointment for the day: blood tests. Mom was in a hurry to get back to the Ronald McDonald House. That was because of Shundiin.

For Thanksgiving, Mom and I had gone to Aunt Sandy's and Uncle Dennis' home for the family get-to-gether, and Shundiin and my cousins came up from Iowa. Shundiin had refused to say goodbye to Mom once again, so Mom decided to take her back with us to Rochester. It was quite a change having her back: she always picked her favorite TV shows to watch and refused to share the remote. Also, she always followed me to the lounge area where I set up my new Xbox.

My cousin Sam had visited Mom and me while on leave from serving in Iraq, and he had bought it for me. The following day, I purchased the perfect game for it at Walmart: *The Lord of the Rings*. Shundiin had never even liked the movies, but she liked watching me play. Surprisingly, it didn't annoy me having her there, like it did before I was sick.

Last time we were in there, something cool had happened. My game character had just defeated a horde of orcs when Shundiin scooted close and whispered: "Somebody's watching us."

Almost expecting an orc or goblin, I turned around to see a boy standing behind us. He was about Shundiin's height, with blond hair. His bright blue eyes stared intensely into the TV screen.

"Wanna play?" I asked, holding my controller out to him.

"This is how to run," I showed him, and he nimbly skipped forward. "And this is how to fight. See?" Looking up, I noticed that he had a Mohawk haircut - or at least he used to before it had grown out.

He caught on to the game quickly. His thumbs moved over the buttons with swift coordination - unlike mine. After a few minutes he handed the controller back to me.

"You're really good!" I told him.

He smiled from ear to ear. But when he stood up, I noticed the other side of his head, and I had to quickly look away so I wouldn't be staring. There was a fresh scar with stitches above his ear.

It wasn't until he had left that I realized who he was. He was the boy Mom had told me about! The boy with the stuffed Charlie Brown. I would never have guessed that he had brain cancer or that he was getting chemo. He looked so healthy and moved so normal.

Mom and I didn't have to wait long in the waiting room. I was wheeled into another area, where a gloved technician sat facing me. Her cold hands rolled up my sleeve. When she couldn't find a spot without any bruises, she lifted up my other sleeve. I was still getting poked multiple times a week, but it still didn't bother me, though the nurses and technicians incessantly apologized. They felt worse about the bruises than I did, so I smiled at them to let them know it was okay.

With my cardboard bowl held against my stomach, I thought about my new friend, and I wondered what type of brain tumor he had. I couldn't help but think that maybe if I had had the same type of tumor that he had, I wouldn't still be feeling nauseous.

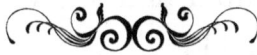

Going Home

I'm going home.

It was Winter Break, and Dad had flown to Minneapolis, then rented a car and driven down to Rochester. He arrived yesterday and had helped out with some last-minute packing. We were only able to leave after Mom's lengthy goodbyes to our friends at the Ronald McDonald House.

I excitedly tapped my feet against the floorboard of the rental car. I would drive back with Dad. Earlier, I had overheard Mom mention to him that we now had a new furnace in the Rothsay home. The money had come from a benefit donation Aunt Vicky had organized in the Hawley community. We would be going back to a toasty, comfy home.

With every bump in the road, I could hear clanking from all the stuff packed into the backseat of the car. There were a lot of Christmas gifts. There had been a huge Christmas celebration in the community room, and Santa had shown up with bags of presents for all the kids.

I did it. Like my cousin Sarah had said: I whooped cancer's butt! I was now starting a new adventure: starting life again back in the normal world.

"The nausea should subside after a while," the neurologist had told me during my last appointment.

Over the next year, I'd be getting an MRI every three months to be sure the cancer wasn't coming back. Then every six months. Then every year. He asked me about my double vision and had me walk a line and do the finger-to-nose test again. First with my right hand, then my left.

"It's been six months since your surgery, and I'm afraid the neurological effects that you still have will remain."

"You mean, forever?" I had asked. He nodded stiffly. My body would never be one-hundred percent the way it was before my surgery. I never would be *all better*. But I didn't feel sorry for myself, and I wasn't afraid.

Tilting my head to the side, I watched the road split into two. I had decided in my heart that it was all okay. I could no longer remember the feeling of having perfect balance and coordination, or being able to tilt my head without seeing double. I had grown used to these things and they were my new normal.

The lasting effects would be a reminder of what I'd gone through, so I could never take my life for granted, or forget for even a day. They would be souvenirs, just like my radiation mask, Zach's bracelet, and my stuffed dragon. I would always remember how blessed I was, and that I was able to make it home.

During the Christmas celebration, the boy with the Mohawk and his mother had sat across the table from us. The moms talked about the effects of the cancer treatments. Besides some minor hearing loss and nausea from the chemo pills, my friend was feeling fine. He was glad that he hadn't lost any of his hair like they had expected. Although my bald patch on the crown of my head had grown to the size of the palm of my hand, I certainly wasn't jealous of him - not one bit.

Earlier, I had overheard a conversation between my mom and his mom. My friend's situation was bleak. The chemo wasn't killing the remaining cancer cells like they had hoped. Just like my situation, a second surgery wasn't an option. His parents were desperately looking into trials and alternative treatments. Worst of all, his tumor had a ninety-eight percent chance of returning.

During the Christmas party, it had been difficult for me to look into his smiling face as he twirled his teddy bear on the table, making it do flips and jump kicks. "Hi-ya!" He brushed his shaggy hair out of his face - almost knocking over his glass of orange juice. His eyes sparkled, and he acted as though he hadn't a care in the world. His parents hadn't told him the prognosis. He obviously didn't know. It had made me feel like crying, so I tried to ignore him and his teddy bear. His family wouldn't be going home for the holidays. And maybe he wouldn't be going home at all.

Watching the passing road signs, I thought about what my next adventure would be. I knew I'd be starting school again next month, but I couldn't help but wonder what would happen in the far away future, when I was grown up.

Maybe I'd show that neurologist I could overcome the neurological effects that I was saddled with. What did I want to be? A surgeon? A nurse? How about a tight-rope walker, after all? Whatever I became, I really wanted to help people and encourage them so they could heal.

On the long highway leading home, I thought about all the kids I had met at Kamp KACE and the Ronald McDonald House. I knew I wasn't the same girl that I was a year ago. It wasn't just my body and my health that were different - I was different on the inside, too.

I now have a new view of life, and I'm unable to take anything for granted. I've also developed a heart that cares deeply for others, even people I hardly know.

These are the souvenirs of my journey.

Acknowledgments

Special Thanks to:

My mom, who has always been my advocate. It was her persistence that led to the doctors finding my tumor, and later, her encouragement to write my story.

My dad, who has been my coach, and who has been a vital part of my learning how to walk and write again. His artwork graces both the cover and interior of this book.

My sister, who has always been so sensitive to all my needs; who pushed me about in my wheelchair after my surgery, and who to this day, is always there to hold my arm when I walk up or down steps.

The Baileys: Cousin Jennifer and her husband, Kendall, for taking my sister into their home for three months while I was receiving radiation treatments.

My Aunt Vicky, who organized community benefits to help support my mother and me; who bought me a new (and very comfortable) bed for my recovery, and also bought me a replica stuffed dragon when my original broke its wings.

Sandy, Dennis, Tom and Erica Jancik. Bruce, Debra and Marcia Hill, and extended family: Tish and Andy Bergan, Carol Knight and Barb Ginsky, for all the hospital visits, gifts and loving support.

AJ, Ariel, Lina, Sammii, Linda, and Jasmin, for being my friends extraordinaire.

Rothsay, Fergus Falls and Hawley communities for the meals and auction benefits.

Rothsay Public School Principal, Mary Donahue Stetz, and teachers: Mrs. Brandt, Mrs. Krueger, Mrs. Peterson, Mrs. Tillman and Mrs. Hovland, for their support and patience. My fifth grade teacher in Hawley, Mr. Lofgren, for always being so kind.

My teachers at Qingdao International School of Shandong Province, for their academic support and care.

Mr. Fischmann, Director of QISS, and his wife, Kathy, for their encouragement and love.

Ms. Cynthia Fernandes, teacher and friend, who believed in me and helped me to believe in myself.

My doctors: Dr. Samira H. El-Zind, Dr. Raffel, Dr. Nash and Dr. Wang, who literally saved my life.

All the wonderful, caring individuals at Kamp KACE in Fargo, ND, and The Ronald McDonald House Charities in Rochester, MN.

Last but certainly not least: Ms. Shelley Gazy, who meticulously extracted the hidden errors during the final editing of this book.

www.ingramcontent.com/pod-product-compliance
Lightning Source LLC
Chambersburg PA
CBHW070933030426
42336CB00014BA/2656